The Ethics of Psychoanalysis

The Ethics

of

Psychoanalysis

THE THEORY AND METHOD OF
AUTONOMOUS PSYCHOTHERAPY

Thomas Szasz

SYRACUSE UNIVERSITY PRESS

Copyright © 1965, 1974, 1988 by Thomas Szasz
All Rights Reserved

Syracuse University Press Edition 1988
97 96 95   6 5 4 3 2

The paper used in this publication meets the minimum requirements of
American National Standard for Information Sciences—Permanence of
Paper for Printed Library Materials, ANSI Z39.48-1984. ∞™

Library of Congress Cataloging-in-Publication Data

Szasz, Thomas Stephen, 1920–
    The ethics of psychoanalysis.

    Reprint. Originally published: New York:
Macmillan, 1965.
    Includes index.
    1. Psychoanalysis. 2. Antipsychiatry. I. Title.
RC504.S93 1988   616.89′17   88-31857
ISBN 0-8156-0229-4

DESIGNED BY LORETTA LI
Manufactured in the United States of America

I have been writing and speaking what were once called novelties, for twenty-five or thirty years, and have not now one disciple. Why? Not that what I said was not true; not that it has not found intelligent receivers, but because it did not go from any wish in me to bring men to me, but to themselves. . . . This is my boast, that I have no school follower. I should account it a measure of the impurity of insight, if it did not create independence.

Ralph Waldo Emerson,
"Journal L"

. . . the patient should be educated to liberate and fulfill his own nature, not to resemble ourselves.   Sigmund Freud,
"Lines of Advance in
Psycho-Analytic Therapy"

. . . the aim of a life can only be to increase the sum of freedom and responsibility to be found in every man and in the world. It cannot, under any circumstances, be to reduce or suppress that freedom, even temporarily.   Albert Camus,
"The Wager of Our Generation"

Contents

Preface

EVERY BOOK written out of a strong urge to say something about a particular subject, like every child conceived out of an intense desire to be a parent, evokes a powerful feeling of pride and affection in its author. This, at any rate, is how I feel about my books, not to mention my children. However, while a parent is expected to be impartial toward his children, no similar expectation constrains an author from preferring one of his books to another. And so it is with *The Ethics of Psychoanalysis*, which is among my favorites. A word about the circumstances in which it was written may explain why this is so.

The Myth of Mental Illness and *Law, Liberty, and Psychiatry*, published in 1961 and 1963, quickly stamped me as a critic of psychiatry.[1] This characterization—accurate but incomplete—made me realize (as my friends kept telling me) that people could easily get the impression that I am against anything and everything psychiatric or psychoanalytic. This is not so. I have always considered a decent dialogue between a troubled person and a mental healer (now called "psychotherapy") to be a worthwhile, indeed an important, human service. Probably because my own inclinations and the urgings of friends coincided so harmoniously in motivating me to write down how I "worked" with my "patients," the result was the draft of a manuscript that was completed in six weeks and required only minor revisions.

Although *The Ethics of Psychoanalysis* is not a critique of any particular psychoanalytic or psychotherapeutic idea or intervention, it has alienated me not only from psychiatry but also from psycho-analysis perhaps even more radically than did *The Myth of Mental Illness*. In retrospect, this is not surprising. In 1965, it was an unexpected bonus.

The reader might wonder how or why this could be so, since the word *psychoanalysis* forms a part of the book's title. That may, indeed, be misleading. However, I have a strong disinclination to coin neologisms. In writing this book, I therefore used the familiar psychoanalytic-psychotherapeutic vocabulary to describe a some-what unfamiliar psychotherapeutic arrangement and style.

In my role as a psychotherapist (I continue to use this misleading word for the sake of convenience) I strive to establish certain *mini-mal* conditions in my relationship with my patients, without which I believe I cannot, in the long run, be of help to them. The under-lying rationale for these conditions rests on the premise that both the patient and I must retain our autonomy vis-à-vis each other as well as our responsibility for our respective behaviors. It follows that I must not have any direct influence on, or power over, the patient's life outside the consulting room, and neither must he over mine. Accordingly, many of the practices psychoanalysts engage in —such as child analysis, training analysis, prescribing drugs,[2] hos-pitalizing the patient, communicating with the patient's spouse— are incompatible with the minimal conditions I have set forth. Furthermore, it is a fundamental premise of my approach that the so-called patient is not sick in any medically meaningful sense of that term, and that the psychoanalyst/psychotherapist is not treating the patient in any medically meaningful sense of that term.

Not that Freud himself didn't recognize, or even pay lip service to, these same basic principles. For example, he knew that his patients were not sick: ". . . just let all the millionairesses stay crazy, they don't have anything else to do," wrote his daughter, Anna, to him in 1922;[3] and that his contacts with his patients did not constitute bona fide treatments: "talking people into and out of things—which is what my occupation consists in," is the way he described his work in 1888 in a letter to Wilhelm Fliess.[4] Moreover, in one of his most important essays, Freud emphasized that psychoanalysis is not a medical activity and that its aim is to help the patient achieve personal autonomy:

> I have assumed, that is to say, that psychoanalysis is not a specialized branch of medicine. I cannot see how it is possible to dispute this. . . . Indeed, the words 'secular pastoral worker' might well serve as a general formula for describing the function which the analyst, whether he is a doctor or a layman, has to perform in relation to the public. . . . We do not seek to bring him [the patient] relief by receiving him into the catholic, protestant, or socialist community. We seek rather to enrich him from his own internal sources, by putting at the disposal of his ego those energies which, owing to repression, are inaccessibly confined in his unconscious . . .[5]

Of course, opposite opinions can easily be found elsewhere in the Freudian corpus. So the question becomes: Who speaks for Freud and psychoanalysis? I have neither the authority nor the desire to speak for either. On the other hand, those who are consumed by this desire and assume that authority repudiate—as, especially in his practice, Freud himself repudiated—the "therapeutic" ends and means I have made my own. Thus, the qualifications I mention in the preface, and others discussed elsewhere in the book, place my approach outside the bounds of psychoanalysis and other recognized methods of psychotherapy.

Consider, in this connection, some of the dramatic differences: Freud—and every psychoanalyst since him, of whatever persuasion —accepted the notions of child analysis and training analysis, as if there could be "analysis" without confidentiality, without contract, even without consent. Then there is Freud's "analysis" of his daughter Anna, which, in my view, is an oxymoron; and his "analysis" of Woodrow Wilson, which is simply character assassination.

In other words, like a Renaissance pope preaching celibacy by day and sleeping with concubines by night, Freud preached strict adherence to "analytic" rules which he unceasingly violated. This sort of hypocrisy, which may well be a requirement for becoming a successful religious leader, sullies anyone who respects others (especially those who seek his help) and must be repudiated by psychotherapists. A decent psychotherapist should set rules only for himself which he then, of course, must follow. If others want to emulate his behavior, that is their affair, not his; how others practice psychotherapy is none of his business (except as an observer of, and commentator on, the human condition).

Indeed, why would a psychotherapist want to formulate rules for other therapists to follow? Of what benefit to him could the successful propagation of such rules be, except to aggrandize him as a great rule-maker? But making rules for others is, par excellence, an enterprise in heteronomy, incompatible with advocating autonomy. Actions, especially in human affairs, have always spoken more clearly than words and always will.

The sort of "mental healing" I have practiced for the past forty years, and describe in this book, is a particular type of human relationship. Every human relationship is, and must be, constrained by certain limits which can be transgressed only at the cost of destroying the relationship. The incest taboo is a classic example. However, this taboo does not render family relationships unspontaneous. On the contrary, it liberates family members to act spontaneously toward one another.

I envision the therapeutic contract—the understanding between patient and therapist of the nature and purpose of their coming together and their mutual respect for its terms—as providing the practical conditions which make the therapeutic encounter possible. Only that much, and no more, can be articulated or specified. Within that space, the relationship between the participants must be as natural, spontaneous, and unrehearsed as is the relationship between other persons who respect (and perhaps are fond of) each other. Accordingly, from such a perspective, there is—there can be—no such thing as a *psychoanalytic technique* or *psychothera-peutic method*. If a therapist is to help a patient in the ways I describe, then his relationship with his client cannot be, and cannot be reduced to, a technique—just as a person's relationship with members of his family or friends cannot be, and cannot be reduced to, a technique.

THOMAS SZASZ

Syracuse, New York
June 1988

Notes

1. Thomas S. Szasz, *The Myth of Mental Illness: Foundations of Theory of Personal Conduct* (New York: Hoeber-Harper, 1961); rev. ed. (New York: Harper & Row, 1974); and *Law, Liberty, and Psychiatry: An Inquiry into the Social Uses of Mental Health Practices* (New York: Macmillan, 1963).

2. See, for example, the "Principles of Ethics for Psychoanalysts" of the American Academy of Psychoanalysis, which states: "To the extent permitted by law, drugs or remedies may be dispensed, supplied or prescribed by the psychoanalyst, provided s/he is legally licensed to do so and such action is appropriate to the treatment and done in the best interest of the patient." *Academy Forum*, 32(Summer 1988):16–17.

3. Anna Freud, Letter to Sigmund Freud, July 20, 1922, Freud Collection, Library of Congress, quoted in Peter Gay, *Freud: A Life for Our Time* (New York: Norton, 1988), p. 438.

4. Sigmund Freud, Letter to Wilhelm Fliess, February 4, 1888, in *The Complete Letters of Sigmund Freud to Wilhelm Fliess, 1887–1904*, Jeffrey Moussaieff Masson, ed. (Cambridge: Harvard University Press, 1985), p. 18.

5. Sigmund Freud, Postscript to "The Question of Lay Analysis" (1927) in *The Complete Psychological Works of Sigmund Freud*, James Strachey et al., eds. (24 vols., London: Hogarth Press, 1959), vol. XX, pp. 252, 255–56.

Preface to the First Edition

PSYCHOTHERAPY IS THE NAME we give to a particular kind of personal influence: by means of communications, one person, identified as "the psychotherapist," exerts an ostensibly therapeutic influence on another, identified as "the patient." It is evident, however, that this process is but a special member of a much larger class—indeed, of a class so vast that virtually all human interactions fall within it. Not only in psychotherapy, but also in countless other situations, such as advertising, education, friendship, and marriage, people influence one another. Who is to say whether such interactions are helpful or harmful, and to whom? The concept of psychotherapy betrays us on this point by prejudging the interaction as "therapeutic" for the patient, in intent or effect or both.

People try to influence one another constantly. This is what makes social life at once cooperative and conflictful. To control and be controlled are the warp and woof of the fabric of human relations. Men crave and resist influencing others and being influenced by them. The question that concerns those interested in psychotherapy is: What kind of influence do psychotherapists exert on their clients?

As a rule, people influence one another to support some values and to oppose others. In the past, values were promoted overtly —for example, chastity, obedience, or thrift. Today, values are more often advocated covertly—for example, the common good, mental health, or welfare. Such words are blanks that may be filled in with any meaning the speaker or listener desires. Herein lies their great value to the demagogue—political or professional. For example, a presidential candidate may talk about restoring the nation's economy to a "healthy" condition, and no one can be sure whether he is promoting fiscal responsibility or deficit financing. Similarly, a psychiatrist may talk about "community mental health," and no one can be sure whether he is promoting individualism or collectivism, autonomy or heteronomy.

Psychotherapists do many things; the professed goal is always to provide "therapy." Often, however, attempts to "treat" a patient are really efforts to convert his conduct from one mode to another. Thus, there are psychiatrists who try to convert unhappily married couples into happily married ones; homosexuals into heterosexuals; criminals into noncriminals; or, in general, mentally sick patients into mentally recovered expatients.

I submit that psychoanalysis cannot be this kind of enterprise. To be sure, the term "psychoanalysis" may be applied to persuasive types of psychotherapies; indeed, each of the procedures mentioned above is often described today as "psychoanalytic" in aim, principle, or method. Even community psychiatry is promoted by persons officially accredited as psychoanalysts.

These developments illustrate and should again remind us that the meaning of a word can be stretched—so far even as to designate the opposite of its original meaning. For example, the Greek word *hairesis*, which means "to make a choice," became the English word "heresy." Similarly, Freud devised a method of psychotherapy to extend the patient's autonomy and named it "psychoanalysis"; today, the same name is applied to procedures which curtail autonomy.

In this book, I propose to describe psychotherapy as social action, not as healing. So conceived, psychoanalytic treatment is characterized by its aim—to increase the patient's knowledge of himself and others and hence his freedom of choice in the conduct of his life; by its method—the analysis of communications, rules, and games; and, lastly, by its social context—a contractual, rather than a "therapeutic," relationship between analyst and analysand.

In sum, I shall attempt to define the nature of psychoanalysis; clarify its limits; and establish its proper relations to other forms of psychotherapy, medicine, ethics, and social science. This is an ambitious aim. But nothing less can suffice in the present stage of psychiatry, in which collectivism, irrationalism, and "medicalism" have not only failed to provide new answers to our problems, but have succeeded in obscuring the old ones.

Yet, only yesterday, Psychoanalysis held high promise for the liberation of Internal Man, as did the Open Society for the liberation of External Man. Both are aspects of modern Rationalism and Individualism. Together they have sought and still seek to nurture the Autonomous Personality and the Free Society. Have they failed? It is too early to tell. The game is not yet over.

Whatever the final outcome, the present score gives us no grounds for optimism. In mid-twentieth-century America, welfare has displaced liberty, and the Autonomous Individual has become the Superfluous Man, the Remnant. The question is: Do we want to, can we, rekindle the flickering flame of individualism? Only to those who do will psychoanalysis as autonomous psychotherapy be of interest and value. Others will either shun it or put it to their own use.

THOMAS S. SZASZ

Syracuse, New York
1965

Acknowledgments

I WISH TO THANK Dr. Kenneth Barney for critical reading of the manuscript and helpful suggestions; Dr. Ronald Leifer for suggestions concerning chapters 2 and 3; Mrs. Arthur Ecker for competent editorial assistance; Mrs. Margaret Bassett for unexcelled secretarial help; and the National Institute of Mental Health, United States Public Health Service, for a research grant (No. MH 07099–01) which partially supported the work for this book.

Parts of Chapter 3 were previously published in the *A.M.A. Archives of General Psychiatry,* Volume 9 (1963); I am grateful to the editor and publisher for permission to reprint and rework the article for this book.

The Ethics of Psychoanalysis

Introduction

PSYCHOANALYTIC TREATMENT is a particular kind of human relationship. Only two people are needed for it—analyst and patient. What do they do and why?

This book is my answer to this question. In my earlier writings, especially in *The Myth of Mental Illness*,* I have tried to dispel the ideas that the person who consults a psychotherapist is "sick" and that the effort to help him conduct himself with more insight, freedom, and self-responsibility is a species of "treatment." Having discarded a misleading medical-therapeutic conceptualization of problems of personal conduct and of psychotherapy, I shall approach the subject of the analytic relationship from a broad psychosocial base, viewing man as a *person* who uses signs, follows rules, and plays games—not as an *organism* that has instincts and needs or as a *patient* who has a disease.

Psychoanalytic treatment—or "the analytic game," as I will often refer to it—may be studied from three points of view.

First, we can observe and describe the experiences of the patient and of the analyst; some of these may be more or less

---

* *The Myth of Mental Illness*, "Foundations of a Theory of Personal Conduct" (New York: Hoeber-Harper, 1961).

typical of the analytic encounter. Many statements about psycho-analytic treatment refer to this aspect of the problem.

Second, we can specify the rules of the analytic game: for example, the requirement that the patient lie on the couch or that the analyst interpret the transference neurosis. If successful, such an account would specify what analysis is (and, by infer-ence, what it is not). But it would not tell us how it feels to be an analyst or analysand any more than the rules of chess tell us how it feels to play a game of chess.

Third, we can discuss the analytic game—its aims, rules, limitations, and so forth. We may speak of this, somewhat loosely, as the theory of analytic treatment or, more precisely, as an account of the metagame of analysis (the rules of analysis specifying the object-game). Such a description will be im-portant; without it, our understanding of the analytic game is incomplete and inadequate. But again we must not expect the theory of analytic therapy to do what it cannot do and was never intended to do: provide access to the experiences of the players.

Clearly, to know what it feels like to play chess, one must play chess. One cannot derive or extract the game experience from the game rules, from descriptions of games played by others, or from theories of the game. The same is true of psycho-analysis. Nevertheless, there has been a persistent expectation—by analysts as well as by those who read them—that it ought to be possible to convey the analytic experience in printed form. But this is impossible. To know what it is like to be analyzed, one must be a patient; to know what it is like to conduct an analysis, one must be an analyst. It is as simple as that.

However, there has been insufficient appreciation of the pos-sibility of fulfilling the other two tasks. Certainly we should be able to describe clearly and simply the game rules that govern the conduct of the analytic players. Yet this has never been done. Usually a few things are said about what is expected of the patient, but not of the therapist. In the words of Fenichel, for

the analyst, "everything is permissible, if only one knows why."*
What could be more absurd? To say that the analyst can do
anything is to assert that he is a player in a game which does
not require him to follow any rules. This is a complete misunderstanding of what analysis is or ought to be. I shall try to
correct this by offering a description of psychoanalytic treatment
as an educational enterprise, comparable to a game, with rules
for each player to follow.

The so-called theory of psychoanalytic treatment has also been
the victim of misunderstanding. Under this heading we often
find authors discussing any problem pertaining to the analytic
encounter, from the patient's psychopathology to reasons for
modifying the analytic rules. But the theory of a game must
provide an explanation of the principles that underlie the rules;
it must also furnish an account of the values which the game
seeks to realize through the prescribed conduct of the players.
The theory of psychoanalytic treatment must therefore clarify
the connection between the aims and values of the game and its
rules. I shall try to present such a theory. It will consist of the
principles of the psychoanalytic relationship and the ethical and
psychological ideas which these principles embody.

Because this is a complex subject; because much has been
written about it; and, lastly, because this volume, though hopefully of interest and value to the general reader, is directed
mainly to persons familiar with the nature of psychotherapy, I
shall proceed in what is logically an inverse order—from the
general to the particular. In Part I, I discuss the problem of the
scientific study of human relations and offer some basic concepts
and principles for the study of the analytic enterprise. In Part
II, I present the principles of psychoanalysis considered as
autonomous psychotherapy. Finally, in Part III, I describe the
rules of the analytic game.

* Otto Fenichel, *Problems of Psychoanalytic Technique*, trans. David
Brunswick (Albany, N.Y.: The Psychoanalytic Quarterly, Inc., 1941), p. 24.

PSYCHOANALYSIS OR AUTONOMOUS PSYCHOTHERAPY?

For many years, I have wrestled with the problem of what to call the sort of psychotherapy I practice and whose theory and method I should now like to place before the reader.

There are two alternatives. On the one hand, I could refer to it simply as "psychoanalysis," because I think that it *is* psychoanalysis. Perhaps Freud and the early Freudians would have agreed. Our aim is the same: to extend the control of the ego over certain areas of the id, as they put it, or to augment the client's capacity for self-determination and making choices, as I prefer to put it. Our methods, too, have much in common; in classical psychoanalysis as well as in autonomous psychotherapy, the therapist's sole task is to "analyze." Hence, were I to give a new name to the therapeutic method I shall describe, I would risk being criticized for using a new word to describe psychoanalysis and thus claiming as mine what in fact belongs to Freud.

Unfortunately, the situation concerning psychoanalysis is more complicated today than it was a few decades ago. Now everyone uses the word "psychoanalysis" to mean whatever he pleases. Thus, were I to assert that the therapy described in this book is psychoanalysis, many analysts would probably repudiate the claim. Psychoanalysis, they might counter, is what they practice, not what I do. Since there is no recognized method for arbitrating such a dispute, who is to say what should be called psychoanalysis and what should not?

Let us assume, however, that my claim is granted. My method of psychotherapy would then be recognized as carrying on the spirit of Freudian psychoanalysis and as representing, perhaps, a reasonable development of it. Hence, it should be called "psychoanalysis." This possibility is also bound to cause trouble, for, if what I do is psychoanalysis, then much of what is now called psychoanalysis is something else.

The second alternative is to call my way of practicing psychotherapy by a new name. I have occasionally done this, referring to it as "autonomous psychotherapy." I chose this expression to indicate the paramount aim of this procedure: preservation and expansion of the client's autonomy. To emphasize the nature of the therapeutic method, rather than its aim, the procedure could also be called "contractual psychotherapy"; the analyst–analysand relationship is determined neither by the patient's "therapeutic needs" nor by the analyst's "therapeutic ambition," but rather by an explicit and mutually accepted set of promises and expectations, which I call "the contract."

The main advantage of giving a new name to the therapy here described is that it would separate it from the many other psychotherapeutic enterprises now called psychoanalysis. If interpretations of behavior, interlaced with the administration of psychic tranquilizers and energizers, is a form of psychoanalysis; if the therapy of psychotic patients, involuntarily hospitalized, is also a form of psychoanalysis; and if the so-called training analysis, characterized by the analyst's active and coercive control of the life of the analysand, is still another form of psychoanalysis—then autonomous psychotherapy is *not* psychoanalysis and ought to be distinguished from it.

The main disadvantage of giving my method of psychotherapy a new name is the one already mentioned: to many it will seem a renaming of what is "really" psychoanalysis. In addition, a new name for a psychotherapeutic procedure tends to imply some radical novelty of method and a promise of exuberant curative powers. But there are no such implications in this case, nor do I make such claims.

I have decided to solve this problem by adopting the following plan: I shall use the terms "psychoanalysis" (or "psychoanalytic treatment") and "autonomous psychotherapy" interchangeably and synonymously. This usage will serve to label, at least provisionally, the particular type of psychotherapy here described; at the same time, it will leave the psychotherapist and social scientist free to decide whether my method needs a new label.

In the past, psychotherapists have frequently exposed their bias toward heteronomous relationships with patients by imposing psychiatric neologisms on their readers. It seems especially appropriate, therefore, that a book on autonomous psychotherapy should leave the reader free to decide whether the author's ideas and methods differ sufficiently from those of his colleagues to justify the use of a new name.

I

THE SCIENTIFIC
STUDY OF
PSYCHOTHERAPY

1

The Psychoanalytic Relationship as a Scientific Problem

THE SUBJECT OF THIS BOOK is the relationship between analyst and analysand. This topic has been called by many names, all more or less misleading. Some analysts refer to it as psychoanalytic treatment, but it is not a treatment. Others call it psychoanalytic technique, but there is no specific technique which the analyst applies to his subject as though he were an object. Still others speak of the psychoanalytic situation, but it is not a single, specific situation, but rather a lengthy, evolving relationship. Actually, I, too, shall use many of these terms, for there is no advantage in coining neologisms if they can be avoided. I use such words as "patient," "therapist," and "treatment" as a matter of convenience, to communicate easily with the reader; it will be obvious, however, that I eschew their medical, psychopathological, and therapeutic connotations.

Before proceeding, it is appropriate to ask: What sort of

enterprise is psychoanalysis? We must realize that the word "psychoanalysis" denotes two fundamentally different endeavors. First, psychoanalysis is a science; since its subject is man and human relations, today it is part of social science. Second, psychoanalysis is a form of psychotherapy, that is, a human relationship characterized by certain aims and rules of conduct; since therapist and patient judge and influence each other and at the same time examine the standards for their judgments and conduct, psychoanalytic therapy is closely related to ethics, politics, and religion. Accordingly, it is fruitless to approach the problems with which psychoanalysis deals and the solutions it offers for them primarily from the point of view of medicine or traditional psychiatry. Psychoanalysis belongs to the history of ideas and to the history of man's relation to his fellow man.

Why Study the Analytic Relationship?

Why study the psychoanalytic situation? According to traditional psychoanalytic opinion, the main reason is that psychoanalytic therapy is the most effective procedure for curing the group of illnesses called "neuroses." If this is so, we fall into our own conceptual trap. Why is this formulation a trap? Because it implies, first, that psychoanalysis is the best treatment for neuroses, but not for such other mental diseases as psychoses, perversions, and addictions, and, second, that psychoanalysis is a form of treatment, comparable to such other treatments as drug therapy, electroshock, and lobotomy. Surely this is no way to begin. Yet, one of the main social justifications of psychoanalysis, especially in the United States, has been its therapeutic usefulness. A celebrated modern book bears the title, *The Medical Value of Psychoanalysis.** But it is unwise to justify psychoanalysis by its *medical* value, which is, I think, scant. If anything, this is its Achilles heel; nor has this gone unrecognized by discerning colleagues, in and out of psychiatry.

* Franz Alexander, *The Medical Value of Psychoanalysis* (New York: Norton, 1932).

Another frequent claim that the study of the psychoanalytic situation is important scientifically is that the analyst possesses a unique tool for investigating the human personality, especially "the unconscious mind." Thus, psychoanalysis is defended, not only as good therapy, but also as effective research. Be that as it may, it is not the reason for my present interest in this subject; nor do I think that therein lies the most important contribution of psychoanalysis to the study of man. Where, then, does its principal value lie? Or, to use the Achillean metaphor, where is our warrior's armor the thickest?

I believe that the main intellectual and scientific value of psychoanalytic treatment lies, like the housewife's key, under the doormat, where no one is apt to look for it, namely, in the kind of model the analytic relationship provides for achieving a better understanding of ethics, politics, and social relations generally. So far as I know, no one has ever suggested this. Therefore, it is appropriate that I support this claim with something more substantial than a personal opinion.

THE INDIVIDUAL, THE GROUP, AND THE PROBLEM OF FREEDOM

The Psychiatric Symptom as Restriction of Freedom

Although the concept of "psychiatric symptom" is generally well enough understood, it is necessary to say a few words about what I shall mean and not mean when I use the expression. In conformity with common usage, I shall speak of "symptoms" to denote ideas, feelings, inclinations, and actions that are considered undesirable, involuntary, or alien. But in whose judgment?

The judgment that conduct is inappropriate and hence a "symptom" may be made by a number of persons: the client himself; his relatives; an expert sympathetic with his desires; an expert openly or covertly antagonistic to him; or, finally, by society in general, through its duly appointed agents (for example, a court psychiatrist). Unfortunately, people tend to use the concept of psychiatric symptom (or diagnosis) without paying much attention to the problem of who judges whom. It is not surprising, then, that an individual frequently considers his own conduct appropriate and "normal" while others consider it inappropriate and a symptom of "mental disease."

In the following discussion, I shall confine myself to those instances in which the client regards some aspect of his own conduct as a psychiatric symptom or at least concurs in such a judgment made by others. In other words, I shall not consider those cases in which some aspect of a person's conduct is labeled a "symptom" by an observer, but is considered satisfactory by the subject.

Keeping in mind, then, that we shall speak of "psychiatric symptoms" only when such categorization of behavior agrees with the subject's own judgment of his conduct, let us ask this question: What distinguishes the varied phenomena that may be classed as psychiatric symptoms? All entail an essential restriction of the patient's freedom to engage in conduct available to others similarly situated in his society.

Phenomenologically, psychiatric symptoms are endlessly diverse. The hysteric is paralyzed; he cannot speak, walk, or write. The phobic cannot engage in certain acts; he must avoid touching various objects, going into the street, or being alone. The obsessive-compulsive is compelled to attend to trivia; he must check and recheck his acts, must think particular thoughts, or perform ritual acts. The hypochondriac must attend to his health; the paranoid, to his persecutory objects; the schizophrenic, to his waking dreams.

The common element in these and other so-called psychiatric symptoms is the expression of loss of control or freedom. Each symptom is experienced or defined by the patient as something he cannot help doing or feeling or as something he must do. The alcoholic, for example, asserts that he cannot stop drinking; the habitually tardy person, that he cannot help being late; the volatile person, that he cannot control his temper; the hallucinating person, that he cannot shut out "voices" and "visions"; the depressed person, that he cannot experience pleasure or self-esteem; and so forth.

What matters to us about psychiatric symptoms, then, is that the patient experiences them or defines them as (more or less) involuntary occurrences; furthermore, since he is not free to engage in or refrain from the particular act or experience, he usually claims that he ought not be responsible for it and its consequences. (Later I shall discuss the psychiatric patient who addresses the therapist in the language of excuses.)

To illuminate the significance of loss of freedom in the psychiatric symptom, let us compare symptoms with habits and work. We shall consider three concrete examples: hypochondriasis, habitual ill temper, and overcommitment to work (for example, by a physician). The hypochondriac makes a career of being sick, the ill-tempered person, of being nasty, and the doctor, of being helpful; they resemble one another in their overcommitment to a particular role. However, these three types of persons may differ in the degree of commitment to their role, that is, in the degree of their freedom to engage in other activities. For example, the hypochondriac is regarded as hypochondriacal to the extent that he feels compelled to ruminate on his ailments or discomforts. In other words, to the extent that he is a "prisoner" of his "symptoms," we judge such a person hypochondriacal or not.

The difference between symptom and habit is largely a matter of convention and judgment: those used to an authoritarian type of family may accept an ill-tempered father as one with a bad habit; those unaccustomed to such a family may see him as a person with a mental sickness. The ill-tempered person himself is likely to consider his behavior beyond his control and hence similar to a symptom.

Finally, we usually regard commitment to work as something freely chosen and voluntary; however, work, too, may be qualified as behavior over which one has no control. Interestingly, overcommitment to work may be either extolled or criticized;

for Albert Schweitzer, it is a response to a "calling," but for the ordinary businessman or physician who overworks, it is "enslavement" to his job.

We must keep in mind that personal conduct is also a form of communication and, as communication, is always qualified as free and voluntary or unfree and involuntary. The possession or lack of freedom of one person has a crucial effect on the degree of liberty of those people with whom he associates. Hence, the concept of liberty is bound to play a significant role in psychiatry and psychotherapy.

Indeed, perhaps the best way to classify psychotherapies is from the point of view of freedom. We may thus distinguish between two groups—one aimed at increasing the patient's personal freedom, the other aimed at diminishing it. Pre-Freudian psychotherapies were characteristically repressive; they tended to abridge the patient's freedom of feeling, thought, and action. Freud's great contribution lies in having laid the foundations for a therapy that seeks to enlarge the patient's choices and hence his freedom and responsibility.

The Idea of Freedom and Psychoanalytic Treatment

Although never clearly articulated, the aim of psychoanalytic treatment was, from the start, to "liberate" the patient. At first, Freud wanted to free the patient from the pathogenic influence of traumatic memories. Of course, this was only freedom from symptoms, in the traditional medical sense. But let us not scoff at it. Even then Freud was trying to free the patient from the burden of bad memories, which is, after all, a sort of *moral* burden. Nor is this idea outdated. Some contemporary workers hold that the psychotherapist ought to do just the opposite. The "bad" memories prove that the patient is "sinful"; hence, he should not be freed from them, but be held more responsible for them than he has been willing to be. Still, the aim as well as the result would be greater moral freedom for him.

Not long after the traumatic-memory phase of psychoanalysis,

Freud developed the view that neurosis is largely a matter of inhibition; the neurotic patient is sick because he is over-socialized. The aim of therapy should be to release some of the inhibitions so that the patient may become more spontaneous and creative—in a word, freer. This idea was prevalent in analytic circles in the 1920's and 1930's. Wilhelm Reich was its main advocate. Although he failed to temper freedom with responsibility, his work, and especially his book *Listen, Little Man!,** is more important in the history of psychoanalysis than many a psychoanalytic classic. Indeed, when ego-analysis was a new discovery, most analysts believed that the aim of analysis was the destruction of the patient's (archaic) superego. Nor was this idea entirely bad. Again, my point is that the analysts were then still engaged in playing the freedom game. They wanted to liberate the patient from the automatic, unconscious influences exerted on him by his infantile introjects or, in plain English, from the ideas that had been drilled into him as a child.

Since Freud's death, the aim of analysis has been to free the patient from the constricting effects of his neurosis (the term "neurosis" meaning unconsciously determined, stereotyped behavior, in contrast to "normal," freely chosen, consciously determined conduct). Again we have the notion of freedom. Actually, the modern psychoanalytic idea of normality is some-how the same as freedom—not, of course, economic or political freedom, but personal freedom. According to this view, neurotic conduct is automatic or habitual, whereas non-neurotic or normal conduct is discriminating and selective.

Although central to the theory of psychoanalytic treatment, the precise meaning or nature of freedom in this context was not made explicit, nor was it articulated into a coherent ethical system. Yet I contend that, as psychotherapy, psychoanalysis is meaningless without an articulated ethic. Herein lies the moral and political and, at the same time, the scientific significance of the psychoanalytic situation; it is a model of the human en-

* Trans. Theodore P. Wolfe, illust. William Steig (New York: Orgone Institute Press, 1948).

counter regulated by the ethics of individualism and personal autonomy. The aim of psychoanalytic treatment is thus comparable to the aim of liberal political reform. The purpose of a democratic constitution is to give a people constrained by an oppressive government greater freedom in their economic, political, and religious conduct. The purpose of psychoanalysis is to give patients constrained by their habitual patterns of action greater freedom in their personal conduct.

Freedom for Whom?

The modern concept of freedom is a complex one. It stems from various sources and reflects the aspirations of men who lived under varying conditions; its aims differ accordingly. Indeed, the concept of freedom may readily assume two meanings almost diametrically opposed to each other. Psychoanalysis and much else in our contemporary society bear witness to our confusion about liberty. By clarifying the role of liberty in psychoanalysis, we may also help to clarify its role in modern politics and sociology.

What are the two major sources of the modern concept of liberty? One is the "Age of Enlightenment": the protagonists— men of high station and exceptional educational attainment; the place—France, England, and the United States; the time—the eighteenth century. The outstanding characteristic of the idea of freedom propounded in this period is that it was *individualistic* and *positive*. To men like Voltaire and Jefferson, liberty was the opportunity of the solitary individual to pursue certain goals: the freedom to inquire, learn, read, think, write, challenge established authority, and to be self-aware. In brief, this is the freedom to be an individuated person, an autonomous, authentic, self-responsible man. Although some of these were defined as freedoms *from* (for example, from theological or government tyranny), they were, in actuality, largely freedoms *for* (for example, self-government for the individual or the nation). In other words, the content of freedom was defined in terms of goals that man must establish for himself. This is the kind of freedom that no one can give another.

There is, however, another kind of freedom; it cannot be truly said that every man must earn it for himself. This sort of freedom issues from another source. Though having its ideological roots in the eighteenth century, in the writings of the political messianists (for example, Rousseau and Saint-Simon), its moving spirits were the political revolutionists of the nineteenth century (for example, Marx and the early communists, Lincoln and the abolitionists). The outstanding characteristic of this idea of freedom is that it is *collectivistic* and *negative*. To avoid misunderstanding, I wish to emphasize that I use these terms here descriptively, not pejoratively. I believe that both kinds of liberty are desirable and necessary. Though I shall be more concerned with individualistic than with collectivistic freedom, I do not wish to promote the one by abjuring the other. The ethic of autonomy, moreover, points to a possible reconciliation of the two.

The aims of collectivistic freedom° are freedom from political oppression; economic exploitation; slavery; colonization; and religious, racial, and political persecution. In brief, this is the freedom of one group, or collective, to enjoy the privileges granted another. To be sure, these notions affect the fate of the individual. Nevertheless, we deal here with the freedom of groups, as *classes* of men—workers, Jews, Negroes. The content of this freedom is stated largely in negative terms, as freedom *from*—usually from harassment by an oppressor group.

Although some men must sometimes fight for these freedoms, we expect a civilized society to bestow them on its citizens; and, in the twentieth century, most people in the Western world have these freedoms without having to work for them. And it is good that they do, for only when all men everywhere are secure in their collective, negative freedoms will they be able, on a

---

° The concept of collectivistic freedom here developed is similar to but not the same as what Comte and others have called "collective freedom." See Mortimer J. Adler, *The Idea of Freedom* (Garden City, N.Y.: Doubleday & Co., 1961), especially Vol. II, pp. 184–222.

larger scale, to pursue individualism and autonomy. Until that time, these values will be threatened by movements that favor collectivistic freedoms, because their protagonists define and regard individualism and autonomy as a guise for the exploitation of the weak. That this identification is false matters little in ideological and political struggles. The fact remains—and let us hope that it proves as stubborn as facts are supposed to be—that individualism and autonomy cannot form the basis of a rigid political ideology; indeed, they are the only effective antidotes to ideological intoxication.

To recapitulate, I have suggested that the modern concept of freedom combines two divergent strains. From the eighteenth-century thinkers and statesmen comes the idea of freedom for the individual; from the nineteenth-century social philosophers and political reformers, the idea of freedom for the group. One is an aristocratic notion; the other, a democratic one. The two often conflict. In this conflict, the psychiatric profession has played and continues to play a crucial role.* What was Freud's position concerning these two kinds of liberty and the struggles between them?

Freud, the Patient, and Society

The thesis that Freud was strongly influenced by the moral and political ideas of both the eighteenth and nineteenth centuries is well established and need not be documented here. He was equally familiar with the writings of the proponents of both individualistic and collectivistic freedom. Which of these values appealed more to Freud, and why? How did he reconcile the conflicts between them?

We know enough about Freud and the early psychoanalytic movement to be fairly certain of several things. First, largely because he was a Jew, Freud felt alienated from the mainstream

---

* See Thomas S. Szasz, *Law, Liberty, and Psychiatry,* "An Inquiry into the Social Uses of Mental Health Practices" (New York: Macmillan, 1963).

of Austrian society. Moreover, when he was a child, middle-class Jews in Vienna placed their hopes in education, not in Zionism. Hence, Freud was more interested in individual than in group freedom. At the same time, his concepts of the good family and the good state were based on what he knew from experience, rather than on what he read or hoped for; thus his ultraconservative espousal of benevolent patriarchy, both in the family and in government.

Accordingly, Freud combined in his personality the values of conservative paternalism and liberal individualism. This manifested itself in many inconsistencies in his personal and social behavior. It also explains the fact that some condemn Freud as authoritarian and repressive, whereas others praise him as the embodiment of laissez-faire liberalism. In fact, he seems to have been both. But we are not primarily interested here in Freud's personality, though it is important as background. We are interested mainly in Freud's attitude toward the patient and society in the psychoanalytic treatment situation. In the beginning, his stand was relatively unambiguous; but, in the long run, it was too ambiguous.

By the time Freud became a physician, two roles had been established for the psychiatrist. They are still widely accepted. One is the role of society's agent; the state-hospital psychiatrist, while appearing to minister to the patient, actually protects society from the patient. The other is the role of everyone's agent and of no one's; an arbiter of the conflicts between patient and family, patient and employer, and so forth, such a psychiatrist's allegiance is to whomever pays him. Freud refused to play either of these roles. Instead he created a new one—agent of the patient. In my opinion, this is his greatest contribution to psychiatry.

I believe that Freud chose this course because there was a kind of double identification between himself and the mental patient. In the suffering mental patient, Freud saw himself as an oppressed Jew and as an inhibited neurotic. To document these ideas would lead us too far afield. Let it suffice to recall that

Freud considered psychoanalysis a "Jewish science" and tried valiantly to disguise this fact. But in a very important sense psychoanalysis *was* a Jewish science, and we stand to lose much by failing to recognize this.* In Emperor Franz Joseph's glorious Vienna, who but a Jew would identify himself with such undesirable people as mental patients? Certainly not the aristocracy, the gentile middle class, or the uneducated poor people.

Great as Freud's contribution was, it was limited in its effect. Although he sided with the patient in his struggles against the forces that constrained him, Freud did not face the crucial ethical and social problems of autonomy versus heteronomy and of individualism versus collectivism. He did not recognize the necessity of making the psychiatrist's position on these matters explicit.

Why Autonomy?

Why do I place so much emphasis on autonomy? What is the special merit of this moral concept? Let us define what we mean by autonomy, and its value will then become evident. Autonomy is a positive concept. It is freedom to develop one's self—to increase one's knowledge, improve one's skills, and achieve responsibility for one's conduct. And it is freedom to lead one's own life, to choose among alternative courses of action so long as no injury to others results.†

In a modern society, based more on contract than on status, the autonomous personality will be socially more competent and useful than its heteronomous counterpart. Moreover, and very significantly, autonomy is the only positive freedom whose realization does not injure others. Other freedoms—for example, to struggle for nationalistic or religious goals—are likely to injure others; indeed, many such goals cannot be pursued mean-

---

* See Robert Seidenberg and Hortence S. Cochrane, *Mind and Destiny*, "A Social Approach to Psychoanalytic Theory" (Syracuse, N.Y.: Syracuse University Press, 1964), pp. 1–2.

† See David Riesman, with Nathan Glazer and Reuel Denney, *The Lonely Crowd*, "A Study of the Changing American Character" [1950], (Garden City, N.Y.: Doubleday Anchor Books, 1954), especially Part III.

ingfully unless there is opposition to them. To be sure, self-development may also "injure" others; the better bricklayer might displace the one who is less proficient.

But there is a radical difference between the injury inflicted on others by an individual who has superior skill and by one who coerces them or harms them bodily. Indeed, to argue that, because of his excellence, the more proficient person harms his less skillful fellows is like accepting the proposition that a sadist is one who refuses to hurt a masochist. Of course it is true that a less proficient person may indeed suffer in a freely competitive society that makes no provisions for the dignified survival of those who, for any number of reasons, fare badly in competition. This is, however, better corrected by rewarding poor players for playing better than by penalizing good players for playing well.*

Because of the intimate, personal relationship between psychotherapist and patient, the concept of freedom is not an abstract, academic issue in analysis. Though at first the analyst occupies a role somewhat external to the analysand's struggles for freedom —from his inhibitions, symptoms, or "internal object"—the situation soon changes. In the first place, the patient has real, extra-analytic relationships—with his mother, father, brother, employer, wife, son, and so forth; second, he has a real relationship with the analyst. In various ways, the analysand is likely to feel constrained and imprisoned, not so much by his "inner personality structure" as by actual persons. The question is: What will be the analyst's attitude toward the people in the patient's life? And, as analyst, what will be his attitude toward the patient? In both ways, the analyst is bound to influence the patient in his search for or avoidance of personal freedom.

If he practices autonomous psychotherapy, the analyst must support the patient's aspirations toward freedom from coercive objects. This does not mean that he must encourage the patient to behave in any particular way—for example, to rebel against

* See Ludwig von Mises, *Human Action,* "A Treatise on Economics" (New Haven: Yale University Press, 1949), and Milton Friedman, *Capitalism and Freedom* (Chicago: University of Chicago Press, 1962).

a domineering parent, spouse, or employer. But it does mean that the analyst must candidly acknowledge and interpret the nature of the patient's significant relationships, leaving him absolute freedom to endure, modify, or sever any given relationship.

The same problem is likely to arise in the analytic situation itself. If the patient feels habitually constrained in his human relationships, he will almost surely also feel constrained by the analyst. This will be an integral part of the analysand's transference neurosis. The reason for it is that we all tend to play the games we are used to playing. Thus, the patient will come to feel that the analyst is constraining him. Herein lies the most critical reason for avoiding all coercion in analysis. Indeed, this is why I insist that analysis cannot be *anything but* autonomous psychotherapy.

If the analyst lays down restrictive rules, as Freud advocated, he cannot show the patient the difference between transference and reality; how can he, when in fact there is no difference? Conversely, if the analytic situation is contractual and free of coercion, the patient will realize it. The analytic relationship will thus not only provide the conditions necessary for a certain kind of learning experience, but will also furnish a model of the autonomous, noncoercive relationship.

The ethic of the analytic relationship is communicated by what actually occurs between analyst and analysand. What distinguishes this enterprise from others is that, although the analyst tries to help his client, he does not "take care of him." The patient takes care of himself. Furthermore, the analysand realizes that he is "expected to recover," not in any medical or psychopathological sense, but in a purely moral sense, by learning more about himself and by assuming greater responsibility for his conduct. He learns that only self-knowledge and responsible commitment and action can set him free. In sum, autonomous psychotherapy is an actual small-scale demonstration of the nature and feasibility of the ethic of autonomy in human relationships.

The analyst conducts himself autonomously and responsibly,

subordinates himself to the terms of a contract regardless of the patient's subsequent conduct, and avoids coercing the patient in any way. Given these conditions, the patient will have an opportunity to free himself of those constraints that prevent him from becoming the autonomous, authentic person he wishes to be.

THE MORAL MANDATE OF PSYCHOANALYSIS

I submit that the original moral mandate of psychoanalysis was to aid in the struggle of the individual patient, not only against his illness, but also against those who, by their conduct, cause him to be ill. An anecdote from Freud's life illustrates and supports this thesis.

One day, Freud relates,° he was asked by his friend and older colleague, Chrobak, to take a patient of his to whom he could not give enough time. When Freud arrived, he found the patient to be suffering from "attacks of meaningless anxiety, [which] could only be soothed by the most precise information about where her doctor was at every moment of the day." Later Chrobak told Freud that the patient's anxiety was due to her being a virgin, although married for eighteen years. The husband was impotent. "In such cases, he [Chrobak] said, there was nothing for a medical man to do but to shield this domestic misfortune with his own reputation and put up with it if people shrugged their shoulders and said of him, 'He is no good if he can't cure her after so many years.' "

In other words, by accepting the wife as a mental patient, the physician buttressed the husband's public image as a normal, competent man. Freud was indignant. Again he was confronted by evidence that his colleagues knew that hysteria was caused by "la chose génitale . . . toujours, toujours," as Charcot put it. "But then why don't they ever say so?" was Freud's inner retort. The reason was obvious: the physicians were not the patients' agents. Thus, why should they have "said so"? It would have

° "On the History of the Psycho-Analytic Movement" [1914], *The Standard Edition of the Complete Psychological Works of Sigmund Freud* XIV (London: Hogarth Press, 1957), 14.

been economically and professionally imprudent for them to do so, and it would be equally so today. I have discussed this problem elsewhere. Here it should suffice to note that no sooner had Freud and the early Freudians staked out their moral claim to a type of psychiatric activity than they turned their backs on it. But perhaps this statement is too severe. There is evidence that they did not realize clearly enough what distinguished their work from the endeavors of other psychiatrists.

At first, psychoanalysts thought that their work with the "unconscious mind" was its distinguishing feature. If so, this could be studied in psychotics locked in mental hospitals or prisoners confined in jails, not only in voluntary patients in the analysts' offices—thus the loss of the moral mandate.

Later, they thought that their work with "transference and resistance" was the distinctive feature. But this, too, could be studied in all kinds of situations—once more, the loss of the moral mandate.

Finally, there was and remains the catastrophe of psychoanalytic training. Senior psychoanalysts, the models of their profession, became training analysts. In this role, they abandoned even the pretense of being the agents of their candidate-patients and, to borrow C. Wright Mills's felicitous expression, became instead cheerful robots in the employ of the analytic power elite. Within a few decades, psychoanalysts have traversed a full cycle. Freud was indignant that the Viennese medical practitioner achieved some of his social success by sacrificing the interests of the hysterical patient; yet, even while he was still alive and with much greater fervor later on, training analysts purchased and continue to purchase professional recognition by jeopardizing the interests of their candidate-patients.

This, in three short paragraphs, is the history of the miscarriage of a liberating idea. However, by correcting our mistakes, it may still be possible to revive psychoanalysis as an individualistic, humanistic psychotherapy. The false medical and instinctual biases of psychoanalysis need no longer concern us. There remain only certain moral-political considerations to clarify.

Psychiatry for the Individual or for the Community?

The distinctive departure which Freud undertook in his psychotherapeutic practice was, as I suggested, to consider himself the patient's agent. In this way, he tried to do what he could for the individual patient and repudiated his obligation to the patient's family and society. Evidently, he felt that he could not do justice to both parties, since the two were so often in conflict. He must also have believed that the family and society were not helpless; if they needed assistance, they would seek and obtain help of their own.

This is, of course, a fundamental tenet of the democratic-liberal ethic and, more especially, of the ethic of autonomy. When two or more parties conflict, their differences should be openly acknowledged; each should have free access to help from his own agents to promote his own interests and welfare; lastly, those involved in the conflict (whether as primary participants or helpers) should not also be its arbiters.

It is not surprising that these principles are completely ignored by all the modern schools of psychiatric treatment; milieu therapy, family therapy, group therapy—these and many other practices attempt to achieve the impossible, that is, to "help" the patient and at the same time "do justice" to his family, friends, employers, and government. I say that this development is not surprising because analysts themselves have failed to hold fast to what I have called their moral mandate. Freud himself spoke hopefully of a future when a demand for "the large-scale application of our therapy will compel us to alloy the pure gold of analysis with the copper of direct suggestion." In this way, a "psychotherapy for the people"—that is to say, for the "poor" and the "uneducated"—will be brought into being which will be suitable "for treating a considerable mass of the population."°

° "Lines of Advance in Psycho-Analytic Therapy" [1919], *The Standard Edition of the Complete Psychological Works of Sigmund Freud*, XVII (London: Hogarth Press, 1955), 167–168.

But what kind of help, or therapy, does a "considerable mass of the population" need?

The poor need jobs and money, not psychoanalysis. The uneducated need knowledge and skills, not psychoanalysis. Furthermore, the poor and the uneducated are also often politically disfranchised and socially oppressed; if this is the case, they need freedom from oppression. The kind of *personal* freedom that psychoanalysis promises can have meaning only for persons who enjoy a large measure of economic, political, and social freedom.

As we move into the second half of the twentieth century, we find psychiatrists trying to obfuscate and even obliterate the conflict between the individual and the group which the early analysts tackled so bravely. The new psychiatric terms—"group psychotherapy," "family therapy," and, most recently, "community psychiatry"—are symptoms of an ominous trend. To be sure, families, groups, and the community—all have the right, in a free society, to advance their values and goals.

But let us not deceive ourselves. Psychiatry has *always* served the interests of families, groups, and the community. When mental patients were exiled to outlying state hospitals, to be warehoused until they died, that was a community enterprise; it was what the community, not the patients, wanted. If, today, the community feels a little more squeamish about such things and wants to have things "taken care of" more elegantly, the fact remains that it is still the will of the community, not of the individual patient, that prevails in such psychiatric enterprises. Behind the unlocked but well-guarded doors of "open hospitals," there are still the involuntary patients, deprived of legal protection and tranquilized into submission. That psychoanalysts do this sort of work and pretend that they are serving the patients' needs has only disguised the problem more effectively; it has not solved it.

Indeed, in the context of the modern welfare state, community psychiatry promises to bring the day nearer when, as someone has so aptly put it, everyone will take care of everyone else, but no one will take care of himself.

2

The Professional Identity

of the Psychotherapist

WHAT KIND OF EXPERT IS THE PSYCHOTHERAPIST?

The Medical Model of Psychotherapy

So long as we apply the conceptual framework of illness and therapy to psychiatry and psychoanalysis, we will regard neuroses and psychoses as diseases and the methods for influencing them as treatments. As physician, the psychiatrist is believed to possess many therapeutic agents and skills, each suited to alleviate a particular ailment. Finally, as in medicine, psychiatric treatment is thought to depend on the nature and cause of the patient's illness.

In keeping with this medical model, it is commonly accepted that various mental diseases require varying methods of treatment. On this point, all modern textbooks of psychiatry and psychoanalysis agree. I reject this view as false; it is the extension of the myth of mental illness into the area of psychotherapy. Let us look at the evidence.

In (nonpsychiatric) medicine, specialization is based mainly on

29

a division of the human body into parts or functions. Thus, there are experts in cardiology, dermatology, gynecology, hematology, internal medicine, neurology, proctology, urology, and so forth. Each specialist treats, as a rule, only patients afflicted with certain diseases; however, he examines and treats the patient with a variety of methods, including drugs, X rays, and surgery. Ostensibly, specialization in psychiatry also rests on a similar basis. But, in fact, it does not.

If the psychiatrist is a medical specialist, which structure or function of the human organism is his domain, his area of special competence? The answer must be: the mind and behavior. But is the "mind" an organ, like the brain or the heart? And is human behavior a "function," like glucose metabolism or hematopoiesis? If we answer these questions affirmatively, we commit ourselves, morally and philosophically, to regarding human beings as machines and therefore to treating persons as things.

Nor should this view be rejected only on ethical grounds. It also happens to be false. "Mind" is an abstraction that helps us to describe certain human experiences, in particular the experience of self-consciousness. Although we have a concept called "mind," it does not follow that there exists a physical object or biological entity whose name it is. To believe so and hence to treat the mind as an organ is to commit a "category error."* To go further than this and consider psychiatry as the study and treatment of "diseased minds" is to transform a relatively simple category mistake into a grand system of category errors.

In brief, then, the psychotherapist observes people, not minds. To be sure, people are often unhappy and unsuccessful; however, if we choose to call them, for this reason, "sick," we use language metaphorically and rhetorically and speak like the poet or the politician, not like the physician or scientist. Accordingly, the psychotherapist does not "treat" mental illness, but relates to and communicates with a fellow human being.

The social realities about psychotherapy are consistent with

* See Gilbert Ryle, *The Concept of Mind* (London: Hutchinson's University Library, 1949).

these views and illustrate, in rather dramatic fashion, that the mythological concepts of contemporary psychiatry lead a life of their own; they are, in other words, useful only as institutional symbols, not as tools.

What is the actual basis of specialization in psychiatry? In contemporary American psychiatry, we find various "schools" of psychiatry and psychotherapy—Freudian, Adlerian, Jungian, client-centered, existential, and so forth. Each is distinguished by the method it uses (and implicitly by the methods it eschews), not by the types of mental illness it treats. Despite the claims of psychiatric ideologists, most psychotherapists become adept at a particular technique. Although their clients have a variety of personal difficulties, all are treated more or less alike. Thus, psychotherapists are—as their name implies—specialists in a method of personal influence. In this respect, they differ from medical specialists who are experts in a particular group of diseases (e.g., the dermatologist or ophthalmologist), but resemble those who are experts in a particular technique (e.g., the roentgenologist or surgeon).

The Psychotherapist as Specialist in a Technique

The thesis that the psychotherapist is a specialist in a technique deserves emphasis. Although this is a simple and noncontroversial proposition, serious commitment to it has far-reaching and unexpected implications.

Although the psychotherapist resembles in some respects experts in other therapeutic techniques, he also differs from them. For example, to be a roentgenologist or surgeon requires not only personal skill but also the use of special equipment (e.g., X-ray machines; radioisotopes; apparatus for anesthesia, cutting, and suturing; and so forth). In brief, these specialists are experts in the use of medical technologies.

If the psychotherapist is also a specialist in a technique, what sort of technique is it? Clearly, his method is wholly nontechnological; he does not use drugs or machines, nor does he make any contact with the body of the patient. Psychotherapeutic techniques utilize three closely related activities: verbal communication; nonverbal communication; and the making or breaking of contracts, or promises. In other words, the psychotherapist's special skills lie in his expertness in conducting his relationship with patients. He uses no special apparatus, unless we conceive of the therapist's personality as equipment. Indeed, this equation of "person" with "apparatus" led Freud to the view that every psychoanalyst should be analyzed. But, if pressed, the analogy between object and person becomes misleading indeed.

THE DILEMMA OF THE NONTECHNOLOGICAL EXPERT

Is the Psychotherapist a Scientist?

Freud maintained that psychoanalysis was a science: as investigation of the human personality, it was pure science; as therapy, applied science. Is this view true or false?

It is difficult to answer this question without first defining the words "science" and "scientific." In our day, these terms have assumed a largely evaluative meaning; when we call something "scientific," we mean that it is accurate, effective, good, honest, rational, or reliable. Concurrently, these terms have lost their substantive meaning. This being the case, it is only to be expected that psychoanalysts claim to be scientists. Every contemporary profession, unless based on art, is said to be based on science. The modern professional is compelled to make this claim, for, if his work were labeled nonscientific (or unscientific), he would be saddled with a value-negative identity. Only when we restore the original meaning of the word "science" and think of it as describing an activity rather than a judgment will it be rational to ask whether the psychoanalyst is a scientist.

Science as the Possession of Instrumental Skills

In general, we consider a person an expert if he is skilled in the use of special instruments or techniques. (I make no distinction here between scientists and technicians.) This is the basis for the fundamental distinction between instrumental and institutional roles and statuses: members of the former group have a special relation to "instruments"; those in the latter, to "institutions." For example, carpenters and neurosurgeons possess instrumental skills and occupy instrumental statuses; kings and priests have no such skills, and their roles are institutional.

This conception of the scientific-technical role leaves the psychoanalytic therapist in a peculiar dilemma. What kind of expert is he? What sort of instrumental skill does he possess? Bacteriologists, chemists, and physicists do not have this problem; they are skilled in the use of special instruments of observation and measurement. Is there anything comparable in the work of the analyst? In my opinion, there is not. The analyst does have special skills, but they are entirely nontechnological; as for special equipment, the analyst needs none and uses none.

Some may object that the analyst's special "tools" are the couch and free association. Since a kind of scientific instrumentality is often attributed to these two features of the analytic procedure, their origins and functions require clarification.

The Historical Origins of the Analytic Setting

The analytic couch is a relic of the days when the psychotherapist impersonated a medical-spiritual healer who cured the patient by putting him into a trance. The patient played the role of sleeper. Since one cannot sleep in the erect position, the hypnotist placed the patient on a couch.

To be sure, Freud found the use of the couch convenient, for it protected him from being stared at by a series of patients, day after day; for this purpose, it is still useful. In addition, Freud also considered the couch useful because he believed that it facilitated the "flow" of free association. I believe, however, that, depending on its meaning to the patient and on whether the analyst *requires* the client to assume a reclining position, the use of the couch may help or hinder free communication between analysand and analyst.

The position of the analyst also stems from the hypnotic situation. The hypnotist stood or sat behind the patient. He would lay his hands on the subject's forehead, or he would use a small object, like a coin or a watch, upon which the subject was invited to fasten his attention. The aim of these maneuvers was to distract the patient from certain stimuli, including the hypnotist's physical appearance, and to help the patient concentrate on the hypnotist's verbal communications. It was necessary, therefore, that the subject be unable to observe the hypnotist. This was achieved partly by instructing the subject to close his eyes and partly by placing him where he could not see the hypnotist. The customary analytic arrangement—the analyst sitting in a low chair behind the head of the couch, so that he cannot be seen by the patient unless he sits up or turns around—is thus another vestige of the hypnotic situation.

The so-called fundamental rule of psychoanalysis—namely, the rule that the patient *must* free associate—also springs from an earlier procedure. Josef Breuer discovered the etiology of hysteria and its cure by listening to the verbal productions of a young woman. He and Freud called this the "cathartic method" to designate the idea that the cure consists of a kind of "cleaning out" of traumatic memories. These noxa, conceived on the analogy of pus, are drained, not through sinuses in the skin, but through words issuing from the patient's mouth.

When Freud first began to work independently, he considered the patient's words the "material" with which the analyst works. Thus, as the hematologist requires his patient to give him blood, the analyst requires his patient to give him words. It is in this way that the free-association rule came into being.

I hope that these comments will help to place certain quasi-instrumental aspects of psychoanalysis in their proper historical perspective. As I shall argue later, the couch and free association are not instruments, nor are they necessary for the conduct of an analysis.

Pseudoinstrumentalism in Psychoanalysis

Unfortunately, the early psychoanalysts never questioned the idea that every respectable medical specialist must be an expert in the use of some special equipment. Freud himself encouraged this notion; he asserted that the psychoanalyst used the couch and free association much as the physician uses the stethoscope and the ophthalmoscope. Though false, this idea has gained wide acceptance. Today, it seems, neither the analysts nor the laity are sure what the couch is—necessary instrument or institutional symbol. Cartoons showing analysts in relation to couches rather than to patients illustrate this point. One I well remember depicts two men with physician's bags looking at a third carrying a couch on his back. The caption: "He's making a house call."

And yet it would be a mistake to blame Freud. Although he advocated using the couch, he did not consider it indispensable. Freud was a fearlessly honest man; he eschewed pretense and gimmickry. But, as psychoanalysis became socially successful and respectable, it succumbed more and more to pseudoinstrumentalism. This has gone so far that today candidates in psychoanalytic institutes, who may be accredited psychiatrists, are often forbidden to put their patients—even their private patients!— on the couch, until the training analyst or education committee grants permission. This, one must surmise, *proves* that the couch is a delicate *instrument*, not unlike the surgeon's scalpel; you would not trust a novice with it.

Unfortunately, the couch and free association were merely the first in a long series of psychodiagnostic and psychotherapeutic pseudoinstruments. Conceiving the person and the body in the same terms, as objects to be probed and cured, psychiatrists and psychologists have devised numerous gimmicks, ostensibly for the diagnosis and treatment of the human personality. Many of these have been widely accepted as bona fide scientific instruments.

Examples of the former are such "diagnostic" instruments as

the Rorschach test (itself devised by a psychoanalytically oriented psychiatrist) and other projective and personality tests; of the latter, such additions to the psychotherapist's and even the psychoanalyst's "therapeutic armamentarium" as hypnoanalysis, narcoanalysis, and the use of modern psychopharmacological substances to "facilitate" psychotherapy. Lastly, pseudoinstrumentation in psychotherapy has reached its pinnacle with recent attempts to use tape recorders, movie cameras, and intricate measurements of physiological processes in both patient and therapist to record the therapeutic interaction.

I submit that all these devices are pseudoinstruments. Their use marks the practice of scientism, not of science. By this I do not mean that, for example, the Rorschach test or the Thematic Apperception Test are useless, but rather that their usefulness is either trivial or immoral.

Many psychological tests—and especially projective tests—are trivial because, regardless of what one person discusses with another, the encounter will be informative for both participants. The question is, therefore, not whether the Rorschach test can be used to elicit information, but whether equally interesting and valid information can be elicited without it, simply by conversing with the client.

The immorality of psychological testing, at least in certain situations, has received adequate attention in recent years.[*] Such testing can have no place in psychoanalytic therapy or even as a preliminary to such therapy. The reason for this is that, to the client, being subjected to psychological testing usually means that his "mind" will be probed; that "information" will be obtained which only the expert can interpret properly; and, finally, that the results of the test will be withheld from him or communicated to him depending on whether, in the judgment of the expert, the information will help or harm him. Thus, regardless

[*] See Martin L. Gross, *The Brain Watchers* (New York: Random House, 1962), and Banesh Hoffman, *The Tyranny of Testing* (New York: Macmillan, 1962).

of whether the client agrees to being tested, the testing situation, like the hypnotic situation, tends to place the tester in the role of expert manipulator and the client in the role of manipulated subject. This type of relationship is, of course, antithetical to the principles and purposes of autonomous psychotherapy.

In my opinion, gadgetry in psychotherapy serves but one purpose—to sanctify as a scientific activity what is felt to be "only" a human encounter. This attitude denigrates both psychotherapy and science. It suggests that many students of man still believe that, to study human beings and their relationships scientifically, they must first of all pretend to be "scientists." But what do we mean when we say that someone is a scientist? Surely we cannot mean that he impersonates one.

The Proper Study of Human Encounters

What, then, is the scientist's first obligation? I have argued that, to be a pure scientist, it is not enough to resemble a physicist or, to be an applied scientist, to resemble a physician. The scientist's overriding duty is to be honest.

Like anything else in the world, human beings and their encounters may be observed accurately or inaccurately and described honestly or fraudulently. In the beginning, psychoanalysis was a serious and successful attempt to make an honest contribution to the scientific study of man. If the psychoanalyst wants to be a scientist, he must continue to be truthful about himself, about what he does, and about why he does it. This implies that the analyst cannot accept anything, especially about the analytic setting, at face value, on Freud's recommendation, or in compliance with the institutional pressures of his profession.

It will be useful to stress further the differences between the physician and the psychiatrist. The physician's task requires that he concern himself with the physical and the causal and that he treat the patient at least partly as an object. The psychiatrist's task requires that he concern himself with the psychological and the existential and that he treat the client as a person. The psychotherapist does not *do* anything *to* the patient, nor does he use any methods *on* him. If we use transitive verbs to describe what goes on between therapist and patient, it is either an error or it is not autonomous psychotherapy. Thus, the psychoanalyst may be said to listen to his patient, to talk to him, or to enter into a certain kind of contractual relationship with him; but the analyst cannot properly be said to treat his patient.

I conclude that the psychoanalyst is an expert, or scientific specialist, even though he has no special equipment. He uses none because he needs none. His special skills are his self-discipline and self-awareness, his critical and inquiring attitude, and his ability to understand and decode the patient's communications and the meaning of his "mental illness."

The analyst must create a formal or professional relationship with his client, as opposed to an informal or friendly one. For this, a professional office is the first and principal requirement. The traditional analytic arrangement—the patient reclining on the couch and the analyst sitting behind him or at least out of his line of vision—may also be useful, but it is not a requisite. As for free association, it is a misleading concept; it is unnecessary for the sorts of thing the patient is expected to reveal about himself.

Because psychoanalytic treatment is an enterprise involving people (and nothing else), we cannot regard the analytic setting as though it were a piece of apparatus used in a physical experiment. In psychiatry, things are simpler than in physics because no special gadgets are needed to make observations; and yet they are also more complicated because situations cannot be judged by their appearances. How, then, ought we to judge them? We must consider not only what they are, but also how they are brought about, by whom, and what they mean to those present. This is especially true in the analytic situation, as we shall see later.

Psychotherapeutic Technique and the Therapist's Personality

Bodily disease is something the patient has, whereas "mental disease" is something he *is* or *does*. If neurosis and psychosis were diseases, like pneumonia or cancer, it should be possible for a person to *have* both a neurosis and a psychosis or to suffer from both disorders simultaneously. But the rules of the standard psychiatric language game make it absurd to assert such a double "diagnosis." Actually, we use the words "neurotic" and "psychotic" to characterize *persons,* not to name diseases. Thus, we cannot say that a person is neurotic and psychotic, just as we cannot say that he is rich and poor. But we can say that a person is neurotic and poor and a good poet or that he is psychotic and rich and a clever politician.

I hold that what is true for neurosis is also true for psychotherapy; in each case, personal conduct must be seen as an expression of the whole self, not as a fragmented bit of behavior separate from and alien to the identity of the actor.

Psychotherapeutic Technique as Personal Characteristic of the Therapist

My thesis is that the practice of analytic technique issues from the personality of the analyst and can never be distinct from it. In this respect, the analyst's technique differs radically from techniques of medical healing, but is similar to such personal habits as honesty and politeness.

The polite person finds it difficult to be rude; the honest person, to lie. Similarly, the psychotherapist's style or technique is a personal characteristic expressive of the sort of person he is; it is not something that he can pick up or discard at will. The psychotherapist who likes to be heteronomous will be more or less directive with all his patients, regardless of what they want or need, whereas the therapist who likes to be autonomous will be more or less analytic and nondirective with all his clients.

In other words, psychotherapeutic technique issues from the personality of the therapist or becomes a part of it. Hence, the therapist can be no more "flexible" about it than about his other personal habits.

This point of view has some surprising implications. If true, the psychotherapist cannot support his frequent claim, namely, that he chooses among various psychotherapeutic techniques depending on the particular diagnosis that he makes of the patient. This is a neat application of the medical model to psychotherapy; for each disease, there is a specific therapy. But, if psychotherapy is what I think it is, then the claim of the general psychotherapist is a pretentious hoax; he cannot diagnose human difficulties in a few interviews, nor can he offer himself as a multipurpose therapeutic instrument.

Do I then flatly deny that some therapists might be able to accommodate themselves to the varying "needs" of different clients and offer widely varying therapies to different patients? I cannot answer this question with a simple Yes or No. Instead, let us first distinguish between pretense and genuineness in human relationships.

If a man is a *person,* he can have only one personality. Or, to put it differently, if a person is himself (as we say), his style of behavior is more or less consistent. (Of course, this is not to say that one's personality cannot change gradually or even abruptly after an existential crisis.) However, although a person can be himself in only one way, he can pretend to be someone else in many ways. Thus, though a man can *have* only one genuine individuality (he may, of course, have none), he can *assume* several others. Indeed, the heteronomous person makes a virtue of being all things to all men; he is a different person with his father, mother, wife, son, employer, and so forth.

Psychotherapeutic Role-Playing as Impersonation

The psychotherapist who claims to practice in a flexible manner, tailoring his therapy to the needs of his patients, does so by assuming a variety of roles. With one patient, he is a magician who hypnotizes; with another, a sympathetic friend who reassures; with a third, a physician who dispenses tranquilizers; with a fourth, a classical analyst who interprets; and so on. Many psychiatrists practice in this manner, and it is possible that they help some of their patients. But the issue of therapeutic efficacy, measured by traditional criteria, is wholly irrelevant to this discussion. The point is that the eclectic psychotherapist is, more often than not, a role-player; he wears a variety of psychotherapeutic mantles, but owns none and is usually truly comfortable in none. Instead of being skilled in a multiplicity of therapeutic techniques, he suffers from what we may consider, after Erikson, "a diffusion of professional identity."[*] In sum, the therapist who tries to be all things to all people may be nothing to himself; he is not "at one" with any particular method of psychotherapy. If he engages in intensive psychotherapy, his patient is likely to discover this.

The Authentic Psychotherapeutic Identity

In contrast to the therapist whose professional identity is diffuse, there is the therapist whose identity is well defined and constant. For our present purposes, it does not matter which type of therapy he practices. What does matter is that it not be a mask or impersonation, but an expression of his real personality; in other words, his therapeutic style and his personal style are basically similar. (This does not mean, of course, that there are not many important differences between the psychoanalyst's relationships with his patients and those with his friends.)

[*] Erik H. Erikson, "The Problem of Ego Identity," *Journal of the American Psychoanalytic Association,* IV (1956), 56–121.

It is pertinent to recall here that Freud abandoned the use of mild faradic currents for treating neurotics, not merely because it was not very effective, but because he could not stand the fraud implicit in it. Similarly, he disliked hypnosis, not only because it did not work well enough, but because he realized that his personality was unsuitable for it; the authoritarian-intrusive role of the hypnotist was not for him. In developing the psychoanalytic method of treatment, Freud followed his own needs, not the needs of his patients; he required a psychotherapeutic method that was uncompromisingly searching and truthful.

Harry Stack Sullivan's modifications of analytic technique reflect his need for a more personal relationship with patients than is possible in analysis. Sullivan was a lonelier and more isolated person than Freud; he used his patients as companions and friends to a greater extent than did Freud or the early Freudians. Again, this does not mean that Sullivan's technique was bad or ineffective (more likely, for many "schizophrenics," just the opposite); it means only that it was not psychoanalytic.

These techniques and a few others are the products of authentic therapeutic identities; they embody clear commitments to particular human values. Like Luther, such psychotherapists as Freud, Adler, and Sullivan said, in effect: "Here I stand. This is how I work and in no other way." In large part, then, psychotherapeutic methods are autobiographical data about the therapists who practice them. So obviously true is this of the therapeutic styles of the three great pioneers—Freud, Adler, and Jung—that one can only wonder why it has been overlooked. But perhaps this phenomenon was not simply missed; it may have been denied to substantiate the idea that clients are sick people whom psychotherapists try to cure by various methods of treatment.*

---

* To my mind, these considerations go far in dispelling the mystery of the successes of many nonanalytic psychotherapists. If authentic, even antianalytic therapists are likely to do better than formally accredited analysts who merely impersonate their therapeutic roles. For a bitingly satirical but well-drawn portrait of the inauthentic psychoanalyst, see Lillian Ross's story of the tribulations of "Dr. Blauberman" in *Vertical and Horizontal* (New York: Simon and Schuster, 1963).

Because of the lingering influence of medical thinking on psychotherapy, clear definitions of psychotherapeutic practice tend to be condemned as unnecessary rigidity. Specific psychotherapeutic techniques are thus often depreciated, even by their originators, because their use is limited. Even Freud was a victim of this kind of thinking; he believed that psychoanalysis was good only for hysterics and some other neurotics, but not for patients suffering from depression or schizophrenia.

But this sort of quasimedical thinking has no place here. The evidence suggests that, when the various forms of psychotherapy are clearly identified, each will appeal to and hence be useful for only certain kinds of *persons.* I am confident that this will be true, not only for psychoanalysis, but for other forms of psychotherapy as well. The scope of a particular psychotherapeutic method is limited, not so much by the nature of the client's "mental disease" as it is by his education, interests, and values. Different *people,* not different mental *diseases,* require differing psychiatric methods. Since psychotherapists cannot adjust their methods to the "needs" of their clients, the only rational solution lies in clearly identifying therapists. Clients will then be able to find therapists whose methods are compatible with their own interests and standards. Without such agreement on minimal ground rules, no authentic psychotherapeutic encounter between client and therapist can take place.

The Autonomous versus the Heteronomous Therapist

There are many psychotherapeutic identities that are authentic, but only one of them is psychoanalytic. What distinguishes this role as a therapeutic identity? Perhaps this question is best answered by contrasting the autonomous therapist with his counterpart, the heteronomous therapist.

The autonomous therapist is, first of all, an inner-directed therapist. He develops a particular professional position and decides what he will and will not do in his relationship with his clients. This decision will not depend primarily on what the patient *wants* nor on what the therapist believes the patient *needs,* but rather on what the therapist, qua therapist, regards as an appropriate professional activity for himself. In a fundamental sense, such a therapist is not for hire; neither with money nor with complaints and suffering can he be bought.

The heteronomous therapist, on the other hand, is other-directed. In this respect, he comes closer to the traditional role expected of a psychiatrist; he is "responsive" to the needs of the patient, his relatives, society—indeed, of everyone. For example, if the patient complains that he is sad, the psychiatrist may respond by giving the patient "antidepressant medication"; if a husband complains that his wife is depressed and may kill herself, the psychiatrist may respond by committing the wife.

A primary duty of the autonomous therapist is to take care of himself; by this I mean that he must protect the integrity of his therapeutic role. If he fails to do this, he cannot "take care" of the patient, to whom he promises to be a particular kind of (contractually reliable) object. As I shall try to show, the client's aspirations toward autonomy can be facilitated by the therapist only if he conducts himself autonomously toward the patient. In this way, he tends to steer, though not force, the patient, too, to behave in an autonomous manner. In brief, the psychotherapist who wishes to practice autonomous therapy cannot seek meaning for his own life through trying to satisfy other people's alleged therapeutic needs.

The heteronomous therapist confronts his patient—and everyone is his "patient," from individuals through families and groups to society as a whole—as though he were saying: "Tell me what ails you. I will take care of it." He offers himself as an omnicompetent therapist. If he does not *know* how to do something, he will at least *try* (unlike some of his "irresponsible" and "rigid" colleagues, who admit to ignorance and helplessness). The heteronomous therapist will thus find his calling in trying to satisfy the "needs" of patients (and others). He is likely to find the meaning of his own life in the actual or alleged needs of those about him.

The main risk in this sort of psychotherapeutic posture is that the therapist will project his own needs onto his patients. When he says, "I will take care of you," he really means, "I hope that you will take care of me." The heteronomous therapist will thus tend to practice anaclitic, not analytic, therapy. His patients are likely to be "very sick" and to "need him" desperately. Overtly, his patients will lean on him; covertly, he will lean on them; actually, they will lean on each other and, like the halt leading the blind, will "treat" each other.

Long ago, Freud noted that a psychoanalyst must not have too passionate a desire to "cure." He was a wise man. The professional identity of the psychoanalyst (or autonomous psychotherapist) is distinguished by the absence of therapeutic zeal or, perhaps more accurately, by a sublimation of therapeutic zeal. His ideal is to change patients only as they desire to change. To the autonomous therapist, it is more important that the patient be free to choose than that he choose to be healthy, wealthy, or wise.

3

Psychoanalytic Treatment

as Education

THE SEMANTICS OF PSYCHOANALYSIS and psychotherapy commit us to the view that the client is a "patient" and the expert helping him, a "therapist." However, the opposite idea, that the client in search of this sort of help is *not* sick and that his helper is *not* a medical therapist, is nearly as old as psychoanalysis. Freud never tired of resisting efforts to assimilate psychoanalysis to a medical psychiatry. His judgment about this was shared, not only by Adler and Jung among the psychoanalytic pioneers, but also by many outstanding psychotherapists who followed them (for example, Wilhelm Reich, Theodor Reik, Erich Fromm, and Rollo May).

Accordingly, the proposition that psychoanalysis is an educational, not a medical, enterprise is not new. In 1919, Freud asserted that the analyst's task was "to bring to the patient's knowledge the unconscious, repressed impulses existing in him";°

° "Lines of Advance in Psycho-Analytic Therapy" [1919], *The Standard Edition of the Complete Psychological Works of Sigmund Freud*, XVII (London: Hogarth Press, 1955), 159.

in 1928, he repeated his "wish to protect analysis from the doctors" (and the priests);° and in 1938, at the end of his life, he wrote: "We [analysts] serve the patient . . . as a teacher and educator."†

If psychoanalysis is not a medical but an educational enterprise, so are other forms of psychotherapy (in which the therapist has no physical contact with the client and uses no drugs). Today, this view is warmly accepted in some quarters and heatedly rejected in others. Behind the scientific problem posed by this distinction lies the problem of institutional loyalties and power, which I shall not consider here. On the basis of evidence and reasoning presented in *The Myth of Mental Illness* and elsewhere,‡ I shall regard psychoanalytic treatment as a form of education.

The question may now be asked: If psychoanalysis is education, what are the similarities between it and other, more familiar, types of educational situations? In this chapter, I shall try to throw light on this question by offering a new view of education and especially of the teaching and learning that characterize various types of psychotherapy. This analysis will be based on the organizational complexity of the educational situation and on the type of influence that the teacher exerts on the student. It will reveal a pattern of increasingly higher levels of educational ("psychotherapeutic") experiences. This classification will differ from those we now use in psychiatry, for the latter are based either on the therapist's intentions (e.g., uncovering, reconstructive, supportive, etc., psychotherapies) or on the material scrutinized in the therapeutic situation (e.g., id, ego, character, etc., analyses).

° *Psychoanalysis and Faith,* "The Letters of Sigmund Freud and Oskar Pfister," ed. Heinrich Meng and Ernest L. Freud, trans. Eric Mosbacher (New York: Basic Books, 1963), p. 126.

† *An Outline of Psychoanalysis* [1938] (New York: Norton, 1949), p. 77.

‡ Thomas S. Szasz, "Human Nature and Psychotherapy," *Comprehensive Psychiatry,* III (1962), 268–283, and "Psychoanalysis and Suggestion," *ibid.,* IV (1963), 271–280.

Hierarchies of Learning

The simplest kind of educational situation is exemplified by giving and receiving advice. For example, if you are in a strange city, you may ask for directions and be given them; or you may ask the French word for "bird" and be told that it is *l'oiseau*.

The characteristics of this type of educational situation, which I call "protoeducation," are:

1. Learning is limited to a specific item. The traveler who receives directions learns nothing about reaching any other part of the city.

2. The student has no effective means of checking the validity of the instruction when he receives it. His choice is limited to accepting or rejecting the advice. If he accepts it, he can test the accuracy of the advice only by following the instructions. He will know that he has been misled only after making a mistake.

The method of teaching and learning increases in complexity when the instructor teaches and the student learns more than advice; and yet, from the information the student acquires, he can derive advice. This sort of education could be called "meta-advice." If you are traveling and want meta-advice, you ask for a map; if you are learning a language, you ask for a dictionary and a grammar book.

The characteristics of this type of educational situation, which I call simply "education," are:

1. Learning is not limited to a particular question or item; instead, if the student knows how to use meta-advice (e.g., how to use a map or a dictionary), he will be able to learn about many things, all belonging in the same logical class (e.g., how to go from any point on the map to any other).

2. The student is better able to gauge the validity of the information so acquired than he can in the situation of protoeducation. If, despite the correct use of a map, it does not yield correct information, he will distrust it the second time; and, if the

error is repeated, he will be even more wary. In brief, the student's confidence in the validity of a map develops over a period of time, through repeated satisfactory use.

Most of the familiar teaching-learning situations fall into these two categories. Indeed, is there such a thing as "metaeducation"? In our example of the student who receives advice and then a dictionary and a grammar, what would he receive or learn in the metaeducational situation? The answer must be: a catalogue or filing system of books and instruction in its use. Should the student want to speak another language or acquire other information, he would not have to ask for advice or wait to be given a dictionary. He would know what to do and how to do it. He would also understand that, to achieve his goal, he must use the method and tools properly. I shall presently show that learning about how one learns—that is, metaeducation—is an important aspect of psychoanalysis.

The characteristics of this type of educational situation—"metaeducation"—are:

1. Learning is not limited to a single class of items. Instead, the metateacher teaches the student how he has learned and what personal and social consequences result from this style of learning. The aim of metaeducation is to teach and learn about teaching and learning.

2. Since the purpose of metaeducation is not to impart factual information, the truth or falsity of the teacher's communications is not a significant consideration. The teacher's task is to help the student to acquire a metaeducational perspective toward himself. Accordingly, his effectiveness must be measured in terms of whether—or, better, to what extent—his student achieves this goal.

An important corollary of these three educational transactions remains to be noted. In each, the educator (therapist) communicates on two levels: explicitly, he conveys informational content; implicitly, he imparts a method of learning. In the case of protoeducation, the teacher provides advice and encourages the student to learn by asking for guidance; in education, he provides a body of knowledge and teaches the student to learn through a method of self-help; finally, in metaeducation, he provides a system for organizing knowledge and encourages the student to use a more autonomous and critical method of learning.

LEARNING, PSYCHOTHERAPY, AND PSYCHOANALYSIS

Let us now apply the concepts of protoeducation, education, and metaeducation to various types of psychotherapy.

There have always been people who say that all psychotherapy, including psychoanalysis, is suggestion. If by this they mean the giving and getting of advice (or protoeducation), their perspective on psychotherapy is limited. This view is so simple and patently false that it does not deserve serious consideration.

Many psychiatrists and psychologists have held that psychoanalytic treatment is a more sophisticated sort of education; the patient is not given advice, but is taught certain things about himself which he did not know (e.g., about his unconscious, his Oedipus complex, etc.). This was essentially Freud's view. So far as it goes, it is sound; but it does not go far enough.

My main objection to this view is that it holds—I think incorrectly—that the psychoanalyst is a teacher more or less like other teachers, differing only in the subject he teaches. According to classical analysis, he teaches the patient about his early family situation, the Oedipus complex, infantile sexuality, dreams, transference, and resistance. According to Sullivan, he teaches about the history and vicissitudes of interpersonal relations. Were the analyst to perform only these functions, his role would not differ greatly from that of other teachers.

Let us focus here on the differences, rather than on the similarities, between the psychoanalyst and other teachers. In general, teachers teach so-called subjects, such as history, geography, physics, and so forth, and skills, such as dancing, swimming, driving, and so forth. The analyst, of course, does both; he teaches content, as mentioned above, and he cannot help but teach certain skills as well. But this is not all. In my opinion, the analyst's distinctive contribution to the analytic process lies, not so much in what he teaches, but in raising the teaching-learning situation to a new and higher level of discrimination and discourse.

We are now ready to specify the educational processes which distinguish psychoanalysis from other forms of psychotherapy. To begin with, the psychoanalyst eschews giving advice. This is not to say, however, that the analysand makes no use of such learning; he usually does. The analyst's conduct and values may serve as models which the patient may choose to imitate; if he does, he learns from advice. To be sure, this sort of guidance is not presented through verbal direction or exhortation, but by example. Though the analyst must not give advice, he cannot forbid the patient to use his knowledge of the therapist as though it were advice. In analysis, the only proper device for minimizing this sort of learning is to interpret it and its basis to the patient.

Most forms of nonanalytic psychotherapy teach by advice. If the therapist deals with an acute situation and if the therapeutic contact is brief, this might be legitimate, just as it is reasonable to direct a traveler changing trains in a large city from one station to another. Should the stranger decide to stay for a while, however, and wish to become independent of seeking repeated advice, it would be best to give him a map and, if necessary, teach him to use it. Similarly, helping a patient learn by psycho-therapeutic education (i.e., meta-advice) eliminates his need for repeated advice. This is what makes education useful to the patient who wants to be emancipated from anaclitic relation-ships—and threatening to the therapist who wishes to foster such relationships.

Education, in this special sense, means meta-advice. Much of the teaching and learning in analysis belongs in this class. For example, through the analyst's decoding of the patient's symptoms and dreams, the patient learns about his unacknowledged ("un-conscious") concerns and inclinations; and, through the interpretation of his transferences, the patient obtains an inventory of his major interpersonal strategies, their origins, and aims. In all these ways, the analytic teacher (therapist) gives more to his student (patient) than does the therapist who gives advice. And yet, in a sense, he also gives less, for he requires the student to work his own way from meta-advice to advice.

Psychoanalytic insight or understanding may be put to various uses; the choice rests with the patient. Once more, this is like giving a tourist a map of a strange city: the analytic traveler may, with a map, orient himself, but not find out where he *should* go.

A properly conducted analysis—presupposing an analysand interested in this sort of learning and an analyst competent in analyzing—is a dual learning experience; the patient learns both about himself and about self-analysis. Unfortunately, this fact has become obscured in modern psychoanalysis, largely because of the progressive discrediting of the idea of self-analysis. Although the analytic situation and the patient's analytic experience require two persons—an analyst and an analysand—this does not mean that self-analysis is impossible. For example, a person may analyze himself in relation to someone other than the analyst. However, I do not want to digress further on this subject.

Although characteristic of analysis, learning of this type (by education or meta-advice) is not limited to it. Certain professional pursuits, traditionally regarded as sublimations, can afford opportunities for such education. Thus, sexual anxieties and doubts in adolescence may lead to hypochondriasis and the search for advice about imaginary ailments; they may also lead to the choice of medicine as a career. In the latter case, the student will learn, not only about specific sexual facts, but also about sex in a more abstract and complex manner, through anthropology, endocrinology, and psychology.

It now remains for us to clarify the metaeducational elements in psychoanalysis. In my view, the basic operation of psychoanalysis is the sharing of information between the participants. This is, of course, true of all types of psychotherapy. What distinguishes psychoanalysis is that it encompasses all three types of learning and places special emphasis on learning about learning (metaeducation). Other methods of psychotherapy encompass fewer categories or emphasize only one—usually advice (protoeducation). The principal method of psychoanalytic metaeducation is the analysis of the therapeutic situation and of extra-analytic situations in which the patient plays a significant part. Each of these "games" must be scrutinized to lay bare its structure, in other words, to ascertain who makes what rules for whom and why.

THE CONTENT OF PSYCHOANALYTIC TREATMENT

From a theoretical point of view, the form of psychoanalytic treatment is more important than its content. This is because the rules of the analytic game may be stated generally, whereas the moves that players make must be particularized. Despite this, the rules of this game have received much less attention in the psychoanalytic literature than has its content. Conversely, I have placed more emphasis in this book on the strategic behavior of analyst and analysand, the negotiations between them, and the contract to which they commit themselves than on the patient's productions or the analyst's interpretations. Although I have relegated the cognitive content of the analytic relationship to second place, it deserves serious attention.

The History of Psychoanalytic Treatment

Like so much else in psychoanalysis, psychoanalytic treatment can be understood only from the historical point of view. As Freud's work developed, there were changes in his ideas and in those of other therapists about the content of analytic therapy. The result was much confusion and disagreement about what psychoanalysis "really" was or what deserved this name. Indeed, in the early days of psychoanalysis, much factionalism centered on the question of what the psychoanalyst should "teach" his patient.

During the period between the publication of *Studies on Hysteria* and *The Interpretation of Dreams,* Freud was laboring under the influence of hypnosis and the cathartic method. His principal therapeutic aim was to uncover the patient's "traumatic" memories and make them conscious, that is, to help the patient accept them. The rationale of this method lay in the assumption that the patient's neurosis was caused by unconscious traumatic memories whose effect could be dissipated by making them conscious. Furthermore, Freud assumed, on the basis of good evidence, that the traumatic memories were sexual in nature. Hence, during the initial period of psychoanalysis (before 1900), the client's traumatic sexual memories were the main subject of instruction.

This specific and limited topic, which the analyst taught and the analysand learned, grew rapidly in many directions. Freud soon discovered that what he thought were the patient's memories were actually his fantasies. This widened the scope of analytic therapy to include the patient's fantasies as well as his dreams.

Next came the realization that so-called neurotic illness was not a discrete phenomenon, caused by one or more traumatic events in the past, but an aspect of the patient's total personality. Thus, the analysand's entire childhood history, not just parts of it, became significant. At this point, the reconstruction of the childhood neurosis became the major topic of treatment. Nor was this enough. Soon Freud's attention was directed to the difficulties which the patient—or his so-called unconscious defenses—placed before the therapist who was trying to understand the analysand's infantile neurosis. With this in mind, Freud stated that the aim of analytic therapy was to overcome the patient's internal resistances to the treatment. From the initial discovery of the psychoanalytic method, some three decades elapsed before the analysis of transference became the central theme of the analytic situation.

This sketch of the development of Freud's thought reflects the changes in subject matter which the analyst, as teacher, expected the analysand, his student, to learn. How was the analyst to decide which of these topics was important? Which was the most important, if they were not all equally important?

The expanding scope of the subject which the analyst-teacher expected his analysand-student to master resulted in two major developments in psychoanalysis. One was a marked lengthening of the analytic treatment. (By now this inflation of the time investment demanded of the analysand has gone beyond all reasonable limits, but still the end is not in sight.) The other was a luxuriant growth of psychoanalytic factionalism, based largely on divergent views as to what constituted the most important topic for analytic instruction. The history of this factionalism, which is still raging, provides an inventory of the subjects which various analysts considered interesting, important, or indispensable for analysis. We need a perspective on this controversy to understand psychoanalysis as an educational enterprise.

Once the disagreements among Freud, Jung, and Adler were settled, the identity of psychoanalysis as a therapeutic method and profession seemed well established. However, the wide range of topics that could be included in the repertory of the analyst-instructor produced a new series of debates and secessions.

First, there was Sándor Ferenczi, with his idea of abandoning transference-analysis and, indeed, analysis of any kind in favor of dwelling sympathetically on the patient's past disappointments and making heroic efforts to undo them. Then came Otto Rank, with his notion of the trauma of birth and its alleged implications for therapy; then Melanie Klein, with her views about the significance of preverbal memories and the early depressive and paranoid positions; then Harry Stack Sullivan, with his emphasis on the present rather than the past; then Sándor Radó, with his concept of neurosis as biological maladaptation rather than as psychosocial creation; then Franz Alexander, with his new edition of the traumatic theory of neurosis, according to which the patient suffers from various parental attitudes which the analyst must repair with "corrective emotional experiences."

Another, more traditional, way of subdividing the scope of the analyst's subject is by dichotomizing it. We thus have unconscious and conscious materials; id and ego (and superego) materials and their derivatives; drives and defenses; instincts and social influences; and so forth. Some analysts claim that analyzing one member of these pairs is more important than analyzing another or that one should be analyzed before the other. My point is that these emphases all serve to distinguish different types of psychoanalysis, each based on the subject which the therapist considers especially significant for effective therapy.

Whatever theoretical convictions the analyst may have, the analysand's unconscious fictions are of practical significance only insofar as he expresses or communicates them. The patient may do this through complaints, symptoms, dreams, allusions, transferences, nonverbal acts, and his whole life style. Much of the analyst's work consists of attempts to comprehend and decode the patient's disguised communications and of encouraging the patient, by means of the analytic contract, to address the analyst clearly and explicitly in his everyday language and to decode his own concealed messages.

My aim, in presenting this brief historical survey of psychoanalytic treatment, was not to condense into a few pithy phrases the vast bulk of psychoanalytic literature accumulated over the past seventy years. I intended merely to place in proper historical perspective the question, "What does the psychoanalyst teach?", and the many answers to it that have been offered. The expansion of subject matter in analysis is not in itself a bad sign. Since 1900, the scope of such fields as physics and medicine has also broadened. However, there is a difference. In physics and medicine, our values are based on fact and established by practice; we know what is good and bad, what is progress and regress. But in psychiatry, psychotherapy, and, regrettably, even in psychoanalysis, we lack such standards. Thus, we must first establish well-defined criteria for judging psychotherapy. Until we do, we shall not be able to appraise various claims, but will continue to denigrate our opponents by name-calling and to enhance our own position by proselytizing.

To summarize, during the first few decades of its existence, psychoanalysis consisted only of the analysis of reconstructions. Gradually, in the 1920's and more systematically in the 1930's, psychoanalytic treatment came to mean analysis of the transference neurosis. The educational scope of analysis was thus raised to a higher level and included, in addition to the patient's productions, the therapeutic relationship itself. Psychoanalysis need not and indeed cannot stop here. A further extension of its educational scope is inherent in its aims, principles, and spirit. Analytic scrutiny must be turned back on itself; "therapy" must thus include analysis of the analytic situation. Nothing less than this can achieve the classic aim of psychoanalysis—the complete emancipation of the patient from the forces that bind him to the person of the analyst.

The Psychoanalyst as Expert on the "Repressed"

Although the foregoing historical survey may have clarified somewhat the nature of the psychoanalytic dialogue, the question remains: What should be the content of the communications between analysand and analyst? There is no simple answer to this question. The best one can do is to analyze the problem it raises.

I wish to re-emphasize that the content of the therapeutic transaction must be defined largely by the patient. This is true especially at the beginning of the relationship. The client must be free to formulate his reasons for consulting the therapist and the ways in which he expects the therapist to help him. Even as treatment progresses, the therapist should avoid intruding his own interests or theories on the patient (so far as possible) and should let the patient chart his own course.

This does not mean that I advocate a nondirective technique.

The autonomous therapist is not a dummy echoing what the patient says; nor is he a "passive" analyst responding chiefly with "Hm . . . ," "Yes, I understand," "Yes, go on . . . ," or with silence. The analyst—as I understand his task—participates actively and meaningfully in a particular kind of dialogue. After the patient determines the topic, the analyst, though less active than the analysand, is by no means inactive. How does he contribute to the dialogue?

At this point we encounter another familiar aspect of the analyst's function as teacher. I refer to the analyst as a specialist in repressions or in "the unconscious." For example, the patient may be concerned about his relations with his mother and father. He describes his present situation with them and then begins to reminisce about his childhood and his parents' roles in it. By definition, this is the patient's conscious version of his relations with his parents; this is all that he can tell; it is all he knows.

The analyst's task is to listen; but to what? To inconsistencies between what the patient says and how he acts; to unacknowledged feelings and thoughts; to accounts of the patient's relations with persons other than his parents; and to his behavior toward the analyst—to the transference. In all these ways (and in others not mentioned), the analyst tries to transcend the conscious account of the situation presented by the patient and to construct another, less fictional, version of it. The therapist can accomplish this by observing, over long periods and in close detail, the actual games the patient plays, rather than accepting his account of them.

I am describing, of course, what is ordinarily referred to in psychoanalysis as "making the unconscious conscious," that is, replacing the patient's conscious (but "false") constructions of reality with his own unconscious (but "correct") versions of it. I agree with the basic idea of this formulation, but not with the impression that it is likely to create.

Traditional psychoanalytic ideas, framed in terms of id, ego, superego, unconscious, and so forth, create the impression that all the information necessary for a complete analysis is stored *in* the patient. The analyst's task is to "liberate" the information so that the analysand can communicate it to the analyst. Those who hold this view assume that, in addition to conscious conceptions of events, persons, and relationships, people also possess (stored somewhere?) another set or perhaps several other sets of conceptions of the "same" events, persons, and relationships. Like the archaeologist uncovering one city buried under another, the analyst—the expert on "uncovering therapy"—exposes the patient's unconscious affects and memories that have been buried beneath his conscious "rationalizations."

Actually, the situation is different. Like everyone else, the patient lives by what he sincerely believes to be the truth (to simplify this presentation, I shall disregard the patient who lies). He lives according to a more or less fictional view of reality. But so do we all. In many areas of life, the patient who comes for analysis is likely to be no less honest, no less sincere, and no less realistic than most people and may very well be more so.

The point is that both patient and analyst will be or ought to be interested in those aspects of the patient's life which reveal *discrepancies*. These manifest themselves in many ways: by complaints and symptoms and the patient's adaptation to them; by contradictions between statements made at various times; by inconsistencies between words and acts; and so forth. It is at these points that the analyst must enter the dialogue; he challenges the patient's explanations; asks questions; suggests alternative hypotheses to explain the patient's conduct. If these interventions are appropriate and if the client is able to look at himself in a new light, then, by small steps, there will be some change in the patient's personality. He will view himself with new eyes (perhaps at first partly borrowed from the analyst); he will observe new sights; he will change and see himself and others differently. His new vision is what we have been calling his "unconscious." Like most words, it is a good term only if we understand it properly and use it carefully.

What do I mean when I say that the analyst is a specialist who teaches the patient about the "repressed," the "unconscious," the "unacknowledged," and the "inexplicit"? The term "the repressed" denotes an unusual class.* It differs from other kinds of subject matter, such as algebra, ancient history, or Latin. The student's personality does not alter these subjects, although the teacher's personality may cause some variations in them. Practically, however, these subjects consist largely of information *external* to the personality of both student and teacher.

But, in the class of events called "repressions," the content varies with the personality of the student. Not only does the specific subject vary from patient to patient, but also among patients from differing cultural circumstances and social settings. We must remember that repression is something each person does for himself. The subjects to be repressed are, however, determined largely for him by his family and culture. In Victorian Vienna, where Freud made his initial observations, infantile sexuality and, to an extent, even adult sexuality were repressed; a cultivated person was expected to have the appropriate fictions behind which to hide such indelicacies. But other sensitive subjects dealt with dishonestly elsewhere were not subjected to repression in the Vienna of those days, for example, financial chicanery in high government circles or social conflicts among religious or national minority groups.

Repression, then, is a particular form of obedience and hence a result of protoeducation. It is easy to see how the person taught this kind of obedience (the so-called hysteric) could easily be taught to obey the command of another authority (the advice of the suggestive therapist). In a sense, hypnosis is the "logical" therapy of hysteria.

These considerations help to explain why psychoanalysis began as a socially "subversive" enterprise and why, if it is to remain true to its historical and intellectual mandate, must remain so. Its task was, and remains, to "demythologize" personal and social

---

* See Sigmund Freud, "Repression" [1915], *The Standard Edition of the Complete Psychological Works of Sigmund Freud,* XIV (London: Hogarth Press, 1957), 141–158; "The Unconscious" [1915], *ibid.,* pp. 159–215.

fictions. Freud, of course, sought to destroy the Victorian myths of family and sex rampant in his day. Today, in the United States, these are not the main areas shrouded in personal and social repressions; hence, the analyst's attention cannot be directed solely or often even mainly to these subjects.

4

Psychoanalytic Treatment
as a Game

The Game as a Model in Social Science

The game is to modern social science what the solar system was to early atomic physics. In each case, a familiar event or system is used as a model to help us visualize, understand, and deal with a less familiar event or system.

The concepts of "game," "role," "rule," and "strategy" are familiar and have proved their usefulness to the social scientist, whether he be economist, military strategist, or sociologist. Thus far, these concepts have been used much more sparingly by the psychiatrist and the psychotherapist, even though the model of game-playing seems especially well suited for clarifying the relationship between the psychiatric expert and his client. In *The Myth of Mental Illness*, I advanced a theory of personal conduct, including especially so-called abnormal conduct, based on this model. In this book, I wish to do the same for psychoanalytic treatment.

Before proceeding to a discussion of the formal qualities of games and play, let us clarify the technical uses of these words. Of course I do not use the words "game" and "play" in their everyday meaning, denoting amusing, frivolous, or pleasant activities. What matters is not whether a particular activity is painful or pleasurable, but whether it involves rule-following conduct. Since virtually all human behavior—from such solitary pursuits as bird-watching to such mass activities as warfare—involves following rules to attain goals, we may interpret nearly everything that people do as a type of game-playing.

In this way, marriage, business, warfare, and psychiatric treatment may all be considered games. Admittedly, this expands the concept of "game," just as regarding depression, conceit, loneliness, and suicide as diseases expands the concept of "illness." The question—which, as students of psychoanalysis and psychotherapy, we ought to ask ourselves—is this: Which will help us understand the analytic relationship better—the semantics of illness and treatment or the semantics of game-playing? We have tried the former; perhaps now we ought to try the latter.

However, we shall not be able to do so if we condemn the language of game theory out of hand. There is a tendency to do this, not only in psychiatry, but in other branches of social science as well. Thus, the modern student of military strategy is sometimes criticized, not for what he does, but for the language he uses! The semantics of game analysis, according to this view, implies a callous attitude toward violence and suffering and thus promotes international conflict.

The logic of this argument is curious indeed: it holds that, if we refer to war in terms of "butchery" and "slaughter," there will be less of it; but, if we refer to it in terms of "war games" and "minimax strategies," there will be more of it. The fact is that war has been called by many nasty names, but not one has deterred people from engaging in fresh conflicts. Absurd as this argument is, it is dangerous because of its sentimental appeal. The emotional appeal of the words used to describe what people do is especially important and dangerous in the so-called help-ing professions, and nowhere more than in psychiatry.

In the case of psychoanalysis (and psychotherapy) we have the following situations. A client, dissatisfied with his inability to cope with his problems in living, seeks help from an expert trained to assist people desiring such aid. What should we *call* the client and the expert? Shall we call them, respectively, "patient" and "therapist" (or "doctor"); or shall we call them "client" and "game analyst" (or "communications analyst")?

The semantics of medicine immediately covers the relationship between expert and client with a protective shield; the role of therapist is one from which the expert may draw self-esteem, and the role of patient is one from which the client may draw confidence. Thus, the language of medicine imparts a vocabulary to the scientific analysis of psychotherapy which supports the aspirations of the psychotherapist and his client. To be willing to explore the possibilities of game theory in psychotherapy, one must be prepared to relinquish this semantic support.

Because of the important connotative meaning of the words we use to describe the analytic relationship, it may be thought that my use of the vocabulary of game theory implies a frivolous, dehumanized, and nontherapeutic attitude toward the serious problem of so-called mental illness. I reject this charge. Words are cheap. Anyone can claim that he cares for those who suffer and wishes to help them. However, if we are to understand what "mental healers" do, rather than stand in awe before them, we must judge the work of the psychiatrist and the psychotherapist as we do that of everyone else—by what they do, not by what they say they do.

We are now ready to approach the psychoanalytic relationship from the point of view of game theory. In this chapter, I shall try to lay the theoretical groundwork for this approach by ex-amining the nature of games in general and of the "game" of psychoanalytic treatment in particular and by describing briefly two types of persons as psychoanalytic game-players.

The Nature of Games and Play

The formal characteristics of games and play may be summarized as follows:

1. Play is a free and voluntary activity. A player is free to start or stop playing. A game which one would be forced to play would not be "play" (though it might still be described as a special kind of "game").

2. Playing a game is a separate occupation, isolated from the rest of life. There is a special time and place set aside for the game; for example, Saturday afternoon for college football, Las Vegas and Reno for gambling.

3. Play is an activity with an uncertain course and outcome. When the course and outcome of a game are predetermined, we speak of it as having been "fixed."

4. Playing a game is unproductive: it creates neither goods nor other products; it allows only for the exchange of property among the players.

5. Play is governed by rules applicable only to the specific game and differing from the rules of other games and of real life.

6. Play is make-believe: the player is aware of a second reality which sets the game experience apart from the reality of real-life experiences.[*]

These characteristics are purely formal. They tell us nothing about the content of the game. For that, we require an account of the rules of the game and of the conduct of the players. Parts II and III of this volume are intended to supply such an account of the analytic game. As noted before, analyst and analysand

[*] See Roger Callois, *Man, Play, and Games,* trans. Meyer Barash (New York: The Free Press of Glencoe, 1961), pp. 5–10; George H. Mead, *Mind, Self, and Society,* "From the Standpoint of a Social Behaviorist," ed. Charles W. Morris (Chicago: University of Chicago Press, 1934); Jean Piaget, *Play, Dreams, and Imitation in Childhood,* trans. F. M. Hodgson (London: William Heinemann, 1951); Thomas S. Szasz, *The Myth of Mental Illness,* "Foundations of a Theory of Personal Conduct" (New York. Hoeber-Harper, 1961), Part V.

do not play symmetrical roles in this game; the two are not "players" in the same sense. How do their formal roles, as game-players, differ?

A Game-Model Analysis of Autonomous Psychotherapy

The Analysand "Plays"—the Analyst "Works"

A game-model analysis of autonomous psychotherapy highlights the differences between the patient's activity and the therapist's. Only for the patient is psychoanalysis a game (as defined above); for the therapist, it is an occupation. This is as it should be. However, there is a hazard in this imbalance; the therapist may resent the patient's less constrained position and may try to deprive him of some of his freedom. This is probably why, of the large amount of psychotherapy practiced, so little is autonomous.

In autonomous psychotherapy, the roles of patient and analyst differ as follows:

1. Only the patient is free to play or not play. Once the therapist agrees to the contract, he must remain available to the patient. In a wider sense, too, the patient enjoys a larger degree of freedom. He may or may not choose to undertake an analysis; he may prefer some other type of help or no help at all. The analyst, however, can relinquish analysis only by changing his occupation (or by redefining "psychoanalysis"). His position is comparable to that of the croupier at the roulette table: he works at "playing roulette" while the customer plays at it.

2. Psychoanalysis is an activity separate from real life only for the patient, not for the analyst. The analysand spends only some four hours a week at analysis, the analyst forty or more. The therapist's office is separated from the patient's real-life space, but not from his own; indeed, the therapist may spend more time in his office than anywhere else.

3. The outcome of the analytic game is more uncertain for

the patient than for the analyst. The analysand tries to achieve a personal self-transformation; the analyst, to earn a living.

4. The analytic situation has a make-believe quality only for the patient. As mentioned above, this is because the patient "plays," whereas the analyst "works."

5. The analyst is compensated for all this by the economics of the situation; the money flows in one direction only—from patient to therapist. Unlike ordinary games, psychoanalysis is not merely economically unproductive for the patient, but actually costly; for the therapist, it is a source of professional income.

The Typical "Modifications" of Psychoanalysis

Comparing psychoanalytic treatment to a game permits us to see how analysis has been changed and deformed. Some of these modifications are the nuclei for new schools of psychotherapy; others, though less professionalized and systematized, are nonetheless important.

1. The patient's freedom in the therapy game may be curtailed or abolished. He may be forced to begin or continue therapy in various ways—in extreme cases, by an order issued by a judge. As coerced play ceases to be play, coerced psychotherapy ceases to be autonomous and analytic.

2. The separation between the patient's psychotherapy and his extratherapeutic life may become blurred or abolished. This is usually caused by the therapist's intrusion into the patient's extratherapeutic life. It is the autonomous psychotherapist's responsibility to keep an impenetrable wall between the therapeutic situation and the patient's real life. This wall may be breached in many ways, most commonly by seeing the patient in the hospital or the home; interviewing his relatives; communicating about him with his employer, friend, or others with whom he has a significant relationship; lending him or borrowing money or other objects from him; and so forth. To the extent that the demarcation between psychotherapy and real life is

obscured for the patient, his therapy ceases to be autonomous and analytic.

3. The outcome of psychotherapy, like that of ordinary games, is uncertain. In games, uncertainty of outcome is a corollary of the players' freedom; we can eliminate uncertainty only by controlling the behavior of the players. Similarly, the outcome of psychoanalysis, as a venture in the client's personal self-transformation, is bound to be uncertain for both patient and therapist. If the patient cannot bear this, he will ask the therapist for direction and reassurance.. Should the therapist comply and try to diminish the patient's anxiety about this sort of uncertainty, he will exert an influence antithetical to the aim of autonomous psychotherapy. Such reassurance can be purchased only at the cost of curtailing personal choice and responsibility; the patient seeking autonomous psychotherapy should not have to pay this price for what he wants, and the autonomous psychotherapist should not sell this sort of help.

Often the therapist cannot bear the uncertainties inherent in autonomous psychotherapy. He may therefore impose certain rules of conduct on the patient. However, in proportion as the therapist gains control of the patient's behavior and makes his conduct more predictable, the therapeutic encounter ceases to be autonomous and analytic.

4. The separation between play and real life is mirrored by the twofold experience of reality: the primary reality of everyday life and the secondary reality of play. The separation between the two may break down, for example when a person becomes "addicted" to gambling and invests all his interest, time, and money in it. For such a person, the secondary reality of play becomes the primary reality of his life.

There is a similar separation between a patient's therapeutic experience and his extra-analytic life. Psychoanalysis does have— and, up to a point, should have—a quality of make-believe or unreality for the patient. This is inherent in the fact that the rules of conduct in the analyst's office differ from those outside his office. As mentioned above, this separation may sometimes be broken down. If it is, the therapeutic experience loses for the patient its quality of secondary reality. The therapeutic relationship then becomes more interesting and important to the patient than everything else in his extratherapeutic life. The aims of autonomous psychotherapy are thus defeated. To be sure, such therapy may "help" the patient, but is neither autonomous nor analytic.

5. This review of the various "modifications" of psychoanalysis points up the significance of the money transaction in this type of therapy. If the analyst conducts himself autonomously and refrains from infringing on the patient's freedom in the therapeutic game, he will forgo the main psychological compensations of "helpers," namely, the right and the power to control their "wards." Thus, the autonomous psychotherapist provides his client with freedom to explore and master his life problems. The patient should pay the analyst for this. Although the analyst derives certain noneconomic satisfaction from analytic work,* it is difficult to see how autonomous psychotherapy could be conducted without the patient's paying the analyst for his services.

What Sort of Game Is Psychoanalysis?

The suggestion that we view psychoanalysis as a game is more like offering a promise than like fulfilling one. There are many kinds of games; which kind is psychoanalysis?

Game theorists usually distinguish three basic types of game: games of chance, of skill, and of strategy. Each type may exist in pure form or be mixed with elements of another type. For example, tossing coins is a game of pure chance. Complex card games like bridge combine elements of chance and strategy. Athletic contests are examples of games of skill; these rarely come in pure form. The classic example of a game of pure strategy is chess.

---

* Thomas S. Szasz, "On the Experiences of the Analyst in the Psychoanalytic Situation," *Journal of the American Psychoanalytic Association*, 4 (1956), 197–223.

Chess, considered the "royal game" throughout the civilized world, has served as the paradigm game for the game theorist. However, chess is a particular kind of human enterprise: two persons are locked in what is called "pure conflict"; what is good for one player is bad for the other; one wins and the other loses. Thus, chess is an example of a zero-sum game. This means that the sum of the "payoffs" for the two players is zero. Undoubtedly the elegance of chess and its appeal to the intellect lie in these qualities. Luck plays no role; each move is decisive and unambiguous; nothing, save each player's strategy, is uncertain. The outcome, too, is decisive—win, lose, or stalemate.

However beautiful a game chess may be, it is not a good model for many human interactions. As modern students of bargaining have pointed out, most social situations which we seek to understand with the help of game theory are not games of pure conflict. Employer and employee, husband and wife, doctor and patient, analyst and analysand do not have the antithetical goals of two chess-players. Hence, in addition to games of pure conflict, we must also recognize and study games of pure collaboration and those of mixed motives.*

In a game of pure collaboration, the players have identical preferences about the outcome. They win together or lose together; this is the non–zero-sum game. In bridge, for example, the partners individually play a common-interest, non–zero-sum game with each other; as a team, they play a zero-sum, pure-conflict game against their opponents. Thus, we refer to persons playing games of coordination (or cooperation or common interest) as "partners" and to those playing games of conflict as "opponents."

Now that chess is no longer our typical game, we have a richer repertory of concepts about games. Let us apply some of these ideas to the psychoanalytic situation.

Perhaps the first thing we ought to note is that it may be misleading to speak of *a* psychoanalytic situation or *a* psycho-

---

* See Thomas C. Schelling, *The Strategy of Conflict* (Cambridge, Mass.: Harvard University Press, 1960), especially Chapter 4.

analytic game, as if it were a discrete human encounter. It is characteristic of the psychoanalytic relationship that it is not something given, but rather something evolving; it is not one situation, but many.

Initially, the game may well be one of almost pure conflict. The patient may want a magic cure, free of cost and responsibility, whereas the analyst may want to conduct a rational dialogue with a self-responsible client. In actuality, this situation presents no problems. The players can rapidly discover that their interests are antagonistic; unless patient or therapist is looking for trouble, they must either revise and renegotiate their interests or part company.

Later, the game may be one of (almost) pure collaboration; the patient wants to receive, and the analyst wants to provide, analytic help. In actuality, this situation can be closely approximated, provided the analyst and the analysand are successful in negotiating their respective demands and promises.*

The Psychoanalytic Patient as Problem-Solver

How we view individuals seeking (or "in need of") psychotherapy has far-reaching implications for our concept of the client. If we think of these people as patients suffering from an illness which they cannot control (and which may seriously affect their judgment about what is best for them), then getting the proper treatment is a matter of luck. If, however, we think of these people as persons beset with problems in living which they wish to master, then we shall have a different idea of the client. He becomes a more or less self-determining individual who, however much disabled or in pain, has chosen to conduct himself in certain ways; accordingly, we regard his seeking or not seeking psychotherapy (or any other form of psychiatric intervention) as a strategic move in his life game.

Instead of having to grapple with problems of diagnosis or analyzability, we are confronted with the task of distinguishing

* See chapters 5, 6, 10, and 11, *infra.*

among a variety of persons as problem-solvers. Given a group of individuals seeking psychotherapy, are they all equally suitable for and adept at playing the analytic game? Certainly not. Persons vary in their interest in changing their lives through psychotherapy and in their ability to introspect, communicate, assume responsibility, and so forth. Although significant, none of these qualities are suitable for classifying analytic patients.

There is, however, a distinction between two types of problem-solving personality which is relevant here. I offer this analysis here because I believe it useful for understanding the psycho-therapeutic relationship.

Two Classes of Persons: The Seeker and the Avoider

Faced with a conflict, a person may respond in one of two ways; he may seek what he likes or avoid what he dislikes. Though this is an idealized abstraction, people do differ in their tendency to engage in one or another type of conduct.

The seeker goes after what he wants. If he cannot get it, he will seek a subsidiary goal which may enable him to reach his primary goal later; for example, he will save money to make a subsequent purchase possible. The "economic man" of classic economic and political theory who always tries to maximize utility (a positive goal) is such a personality.*

The avoider, on the other hand, moves away from what he does not want. Instead of trying to maximize utility, he attempts to minimize disutility (a negative goal). For example, if a man is compelled to work, he will try to work as little as possible. The seeker is moved by the hope of gain; the avoider, by the fear of loss.

Though probably unaware of this polarity, Freud made his ideal patient the seeker, not the avoider. He assumed that his patient—for example, a hysterical woman—sought a positive goal: instinctual (sexual) gratification. Hence, the therapist's

---

* See Kenneth E. Boulding, *Conflict and Defense,* "A General Theory" (New York: Harper & Brothers, 1962), especially Chapter 5.

task was to clarify the goal and remove the inhibitions that prevented her from attaining it. The whole enterprise was based on the premise that the patient is more interested in obtaining satisfaction than in avoiding painful problems and tasks. A great deal of psychoanalytic theory and practice founders on this point.

The seeker and the avoider confront the analyst with two different problems. I shall describe each, perhaps in slightly exaggerated form, because patients are often motivated by a shifting balance of positive and negative goals. Nevertheless, the following comments accord closely with and are based on my experiences as a psychotherapist.

The Seeker

The seeker regards the analytic enterprise as a means of achieving a particular goal, for example, better self-control, increased ability to work, a happier marriage or divorce. He has a commitment to certain values, formed before he undertakes analysis, and he seeks ways to realize his aspirations.

The analyst and the analytic process may or may not help the seeker. Regardless of the outcome, neither analyst nor analysand will find himself in the sort of difficult situation that the avoider and his therapist often do. Thus, the analyst will not have to face the problem of being confronted with a person who does not really want anything—except peace and quiet, safety and security. And the analysand, if he is a seeker, will not feel compelled to visit an analyst who does not seem to be helping him. Because of his personality, the seeker will tend to persist in efforts to attain his goals, but not necessarily by a single method; if one method fails, he will try another. If a particular analyst fails him, he will try another; and, if analysis itself seems unpromising, he will try other ways of solving his problems.

Because he is freer to avail himself of other means of self-realization, the seeker does not "need" analytic help as much as does the avoider. Paradoxically, however, he is more likely to solicit analytic help—not because he needs it more than the avoider, but because he *is* a seeker. Finally, and for the same reasons, he, not the avoider, is more likely to benefit from analysis or to "recover" from his "neurosis" without any formal therapeutic help. The analyst eager to have therapeutic successes would do well to limit his clientele to seekers. If so selected, however, his patients will not be proper subjects for protracted, economically lucrative analyses, whereas the avoiders often are.

The Avoider

The seeker is like the businessman or entrepreneur whose aim is maximal profits; the avoider, like the employee or laborer whose aim is minimal effort. Because of the nature of so-called psychiatric symptoms, many patients receiving psychotherapy—and most of those who do not want it for themselves but are coerced into it—are motivated largely by the desire to avoid, rather than overcome, problems. For example, the hysteric tries to avoid temptation; the phobic, confrontation with authority; the schizoid, people who will control him; and so forth.

It follows, then, that, though it is the avoider who "really needs" analysis, he is likely to display the same attitude toward analysis as he does toward other things, that is, he will avoid it. Nevertheless, prompted mainly by their suffering, many persons with avoidance-oriented styles of life do solicit psychotherapeutic help. Such a patient and his therapist are likely to assume that modification of the patient's suffering through analytic work will be a worthwhile achievement. Actually, it may not be. (Hence the need for a properly conducted trial period.)

Let me add here that I consider avoiders just as "analyzable" as seekers. The problem is not that they are not analyzable, but that they hope to get something for nothing, or, to put it more technically, that they hope to use autonomous psychotherapy to improve their skills in living heteronomously. This apparent paradox stems from the ambiguity inherent in the words "seeker" and "avoider"; each can be described in terms of the other. Thus, the seeker tries to avoid frustration, ignorance, and lack of mastery; the avoider seeks to attain harmony, peace, and security. Accordingly, avoiders have as much reason to seek analytic help to attain their goals as seekers do to attain theirs.

It is necessary that the analyst recognize this problem and, if appropriate, discuss it with his client. The patient must then grapple with it and solve it to his own satisfaction.

But what exactly is the problem? It is this: if the patient is free to use analysis as he sees fit, he may use it to avoid conflicts and problems, not to solve them; to subjugate himself to the analyst, not to free himself from his internalized oppressors; to minimize pain and effort, not to maximize pleasure and creativity; in brief, he may use analysis to become even more heteronomous, not autonomous.

Patients like this have been a perennial thorn in the side of psychoanalysts. But they need not be. It is not the psycho-analyst's job to change anyone. Freud said this often, but often seemed to forget it. When patients use analysis to avoid problems, they are often labeled "resistant"; when they avoid pain even at the cost of injuring themselves, "masochistic"; and, when they avoid life itself because it is too arduous, "passive." However accurate these labels may be, they do not lessen the problem for either patient or analyst.

As a rule, it requires a long period of analytic work before either analyst or patient can fully grasp the avoidance value of the patient's habitual ("neurotic") life strategies. When they do, several questions arise: How can the avoidance goals of the patient be best attained—through his symptoms and life style or through analysis and a modification of his personality? Should the client supplement his negative goals with some positive ones? Should he try to abandon some of his negative goals?

For the autonomous therapist, the avoider presents a much more difficult problem than does the seeker. The patient's task is also more difficult; however, he also has more to gain than does the seeker. This is because, once avoidance strategies are well established, they are not likely to change "spontaneously." Such life styles are exceedingly stable. Thus, unless the avoider has the good fortune to encounter a competent analyst and the good sense to make use of an analysis, he is not likely to change his personality. The seeker, on the other hand, has many opportunities for personal self-transformation besides psychoanalysis.

What is the analyst's task when confronted by an inveterate avoider? Surely it is no more his job to try to change avoiders to seekers than seekers to avoiders. However, the therapist should recognize and encourage his patient to recognize that analysis is predicated on a philosophy of seeking, rather than of avoiding. They should also realize that, though this value preference is necessary for the analyst, it is not for the patient. The analysand must be free to choose among goals and values. In brief, only the analyst must value autonomy. It is preferable if the patient values it also, but he cannot be required to do so.

The relation between analyst and patient is comparable to that between government and citizen in an ideal open society. In such a society, the individual must be free to abjure liberty; were he not, he would have no liberty to abjure. The government, however, must not be free to choose despotism, regardless of how much its citizens demand it. In brief, the individual may act like a slave, but the government may not act like a tyrant. Similarly, the analysand may act like an avoider, but the analyst must act like a seeker. Needless to say, it is preferable that such value conflicts be minimized. If they are not, the heteronomous citizen will subvert the open society and the heteronomous patient will tend to force his therapist into a complementary, directive-oppressive role. The analyst must resist this temptation, as he must others, without either coercing the patient or dismissing him from therapy.

In principle, autonomous psychotherapy could help a person become a better avoider of life problems than he was before therapy. If his chief aim is to "play it safe," he may use the analytic relationship to improve his skill to live without serious commitment to persons or values. It is also possible that the analysis may undermine this skill. In particular, the patient may realize—and this may come as a shock to him—that, despite successful avoidance of risks and social difficulties, his strategies leave him existentially empty-handed. In addition, exposure to the analytic game may make such a person increasingly unfit to function smoothly in the heteronomous, bureaucratic games in which he had formerly excelled. Sooner or later, such a person may either leave therapy or confront himself with the question: Of what use is an awareness of choices for a person who does not want to make choices?

This is the predicament that faced Adolf Eichmann when Germany was defeated in May 1945. According to Hannah Arendt, this is what he said to himself:

> I sensed I would have to lead a leaderless and difficult individual life, I would receive no directive from anybody, no orders or commands would any longer be issued to me, no pertinent ordinances would be there to consult—in brief, a life never known before lay before me.*

This statement sums up the dilemma of heteronomous man contemplating the possibility of an autonomous existence. The psychoanalyst cannot and need not solve this problem for the patient, but must leave him free either to seek other leaders or to undertake the slow and painful task of learning to stand alone.

* *Eichmann in Jerusalem,* "A Report on the Banality of Evil" (New York: Viking, 1963), p. 28.

II

THE THEORY OF
AUTONOMOUS
PSYCHOTHERAPY

5

The Initial Contact between Patient and Therapist

THE RELATIONSHIP BETWEEN patient and analyst may be divided into four phases: (1) the initial interviews, (2) the trial period, (3) the contractual phase, and (4) the terminal period. In the first phase, client and therapist meet and appraise each other; the patient indicates what he wishes to buy, and the therapist, what he offers to sell. The two parties thus have an opportunity to decide whether they wish to embark on what is traditionally defined as a psychoanalytic procedure. If they do, the trial period begins. The therapeutic relationship may remain in this phase (sometimes for an extended period), be continued into a contractual phase, or be terminated. If analysis progresses to contract, its termination must follow certain rules.

In this chapter, I shall describe, in theoretical terms, the first phase of psychoanalytic treatment.

THE TREATMENT GAME AND THE EDUCATION GAME

The application of the medical-therapeutic frame of reference to psychoanalysis creates difficulties at every point during the analytic relationship. In psychoanalysis, when client and expert first meet, we usually refer to the former as a "patient" and to the latter as a "therapist." Like other therapists, the analyst is expected to make a diagnosis, recommend therapy, and, in some cases, carry out the treatment. It is thus generally accepted that the analyst's initial task is to assess the patient's "psycho-dynamics" and decide whether he is "analyzable." I submit, however, that this is not the analyst's task.

To understand the reasons why patients for autonomous psychotherapy cannot be selected as, say, patients for surgery are, we must compare the patient role to the student role. This will help us to understand the difference between the medical view of patient-selection and the educational view of student-selection (which is actually not a process of selection at all).

The Patient Role and the Student Role

A sick person is a layman. Even a physician, when sick, is expected to behave as though he did not know what was the matter with him. Thus, the sick person, essentially ignorant of the nature of his illness, visits the doctor. The physician, with his special knowledge and skills, makes a diagnosis and carries out the necessary treatment. The patient's part is usually limited to having the right to accept or reject the treatment offered.

If the student is an independent adult (or is permitted to act autonomously), it is he (not someone else, no matter how expert) who establishes the "diagnosis," that is, the problem to be solved. Educational problems, no less than medical, vary greatly. For example, the student may lack medical skills or familiarity with Russian; if he wishes to become a physician or learn Russian, he will study these subjects. Similarly, a person may lack self-understanding and interpersonal skills; his own conduct or the conduct of others may puzzle him and cause him dissatisfaction; to improve his personal well-being, he may choose to learn more about himself and his relations to others. Such a person may seek help from an analyst.

There is another difference between the situation of the medical patient and the self-responsible student; it pertains to the *goals* inherent in the patient and student roles.

The patient is sick and aspires to become healthy. His physician has the same goal, as a rule. This is because the sickness and health of the human body are issues on which there is broad agreement among Western people. Finally, the sick person usually has a personal identity in addition to and independent of his being sick. He goes to the doctor, not to seek a new identity, but to alter certain conditions that interfere with his playing his accustomed social role and hence with his experiencing his accustomed identity.

In contrast, the student is not sick; he is—and I speak here descriptively, not pejoratively—ignorant or unskilled (not totally, of course, for, in actuality, no adult person can be). His naïveté or stupidity involves only certain activities or subjects. A graduate student of physics is ignorant of this science in the sense that he wishes to learn more about it; a medical student is ignorant of medicine in the same sense. But, whereas the sick person is considered ill and is in the patient role because his body functioning deviates from the norm, the student is considered ignorant and is in the student role, not because he deviates from socially accepted norms of education, but because he wants to fulfill a personal aspiration.

Furthermore, there are no norms of education comparable to the widely shared norm of bodily health. For a Greek scholar, education is one thing; for an art historian, another; for a physicist, a third; for an athlete, a fourth; and so on. There are many kinds of knowledge and skill, and each of us may be knowledgeable or skilled in some, but not all. The point is that to select oneself for the student role in a particular subject is, above all else, an *existential choice*. This is partly a judgment about one's self, partly a commitment to self-transformation.

Accordingly, if psychotherapy is a learning process (rather than a process of regaining lost health) and if it involves a transformation of the self (rather than an alteration in the structure or function of the body), we ought to be very clear about *who decides what about whose self-transformation*. Like policemen and judges, psychiatrists are often called on by persons and social agencies who wish another person's self to be transformed. Although the term "psychiatrist" is applied both to the psychiatrist who does this sort of work and to his psychoanalytic colleague, they are engaged in diametrically opposed enterprises. The former treats patients whose personality transformation is desired by others; the latter must limit his contacts to those who desire their own self-transformation.

In my opinion, the analyst has no right to act as though his task were to establish, much less enforce, whether a person should become an analytic patient. His right is limited to refusing to accept anyone he does not wish to treat. He should not, therefore, tell a person seeking analytic help that another kind of treatment would be better for him. If the analyst respects human dignity and self-determination, he must not do this.

In sum, the therapist who wishes to practice autonomous psychotherapy must renounce the role of the psychodiagnostician, for it debases the patient. This does not mean that the therapist must accept everyone who comes to him wanting to be analyzed. It only means that the selective process should be mutual rather than unilateral and autonomous rather than coercive for both participants.

WHO SELECTS WHOM?

This raises the question of the selection of patients for analysis. In the traditional approach, the analyst tries to assess whether the patient is analyzable; he accepts those patients who are and rejects (that is, makes other recommendations to) those who are not. This point of view is incompatible with the principles of autonomous psychotherapy.

The client who seeks help from an analyst is bound to have some doubt. What is wrong with him? Can he be helped? If so, is analysis the sort of help he needs or wants? Does the analyst know his business? The standard analytic procedure, which is modeled on the doctor–patient relationship, tends to cast these doubts into a certain mold; thus, the client is likely to express his fears in the form of two questions (which he may actually ask): "Am I a good patient?" and "Can I be analyzed?" These doubts are often mirrored in the mind of the analyst. He may ask himself: "Is this going to be an easy or a difficult patient?" and "Is this patient analyzable?" If the answer to the second question is No, it often implies that both patient and therapist will have to be satisfied with some inferior kind of therapy. This is a psychological bind that must be avoided. Indeed, these questions are so basic to the analytic encounter that they require further discussion and clarification.

The therapist is a respected authority whom the patient seeks out, pays for his services, and tries to please (and displease). From this arises the problem of the patient's need to be compliant vis-à-vis the therapist. This is directly contrary to the aim of analysis, which is to liberate the patient from intrapersonal, interpersonal, and social oppression. All this is well known. Freud formulated this problem by speaking of the patient's transference to the physician and the analyst's obligation to analyze, rather than exploit, this type of human bondage.

Though this formulation is sound, we should not forget that the psychoanalytic situation plays a crucial role in determining what sort of relationship develops between these two persons and what can and cannot be done with it. Thus, if the analytic setting is oppressive for the patient, if it forces him to submit to unnecessary indignities and humiliations to maintain the relationship with the therapist, then no amount of "analyzing" the transference can liberate the patient. Indeed, such a situation presents him with a kind of double talk (or double bind)—the analyst oppressing the patient by engaging him in an authoritarian-coercive therapeutic situation while "interpreting" his infantile, dependent, or submissive postures toward others.

The question, "Am I a good patient?", is a trap for both patient and therapist. If the analyst suggests an affirmative answer, it means, "Yes, you are a good boy (student, penitent, etc.)," and that the therapist accepts a superior role for himself so that he can legitimately judge the client's conduct in the patient role. If the answer is No, the meaning is the same, but the condemnation is stronger. In either case, the therapist–patient relationship is cast in a superior–inferior polarity. I believe that many psychotherapeutic encounters flounder on this point: The more the client tries to be a "good analytic patient," the more he is destined to fail—whether or not he succeeds in pleasing the therapist.

In such predicaments, there is only one way out, namely, assuming an analytic or logical metaposition toward the problem. The trap must be scrutinized and transcended. Here, again, the proper use of both trial period and contract is important. As it becomes clear what the therapist and client want, it is possible for each to decide whether to engage in analysis with the other. This means that the analyst need not be concerned about whether the patient is a "neurotic" or "borderline psychotic" or whether he is "analyzable."

The problem which these abstractions seek to resolve must be formulated in more practical, operational terms, such as: Does the patient understand what the analyst expects of him? Is he interested in participating in the analytic game? Can he, in fact, participate in it? These questions can be readily answered by gradually making known to the patient the rule requirements of the analytic situation. If the therapist conducts himself in this fashion, the problem of selecting patients for analysis becomes simplified. Instead of having to make profound guesses about the patient's hidden "psychodynamics," the patient's conduct during the initial interviews will settle the question. If the patient does not want analysis or cannot tolerate the conditions which it imposes on him, he will decide not to buy what the analyst sells. This is usually how the selection process works in my hands. I do not really select the patients; they choose or reject me.

THE SIGNIFICANCE OF THE PATIENT'S SELF-SELECTION

If a young man chooses a career in medicine, the ministry, physics, or politics, we are justified in regarding his choice as an expression of who he is and what he wishes to become. Similarly, if a person is beset by problems in living and chooses to consult one type of mental healer rather than another, it is an expression of who he is and what he wishes to become. The psychotherapist cannot evade this problem. He has three choices. First, he may accept the patient's choice as best for the patient. Second, he may appraise the patient as incapable of knowing what he needs and hence prescribe the kind of therapy he ought to have. Third, he may supplement the patient's information about the type of help available and allow him to base new decisions on it. The point is that the therapist cannot *decide* what sort of therapy the patient ought to have (although the patient might like him to do so) and then propose to analyze him.

The autonomous psychotherapist must eschew such heteronomous interventions, for there is no way of judging whether a particular person with problems in living should be "treated" by psychoanalysis, religious counseling, drugs, electric shock, or any of a host of other procedures. The analyst is committed to viewing the patient's decisions, including his choice of therapy, as acts of self-revelation and hence as sources of information about the patient to be "interpreted" to him, rather than as errors to be authoritatively "corrected" by the therapist.

An example will illustrate what I mean. A well-educated young woman is unhappy in her marriage and bored with her role of mother and housewife. She may consult an organic-directive psychiatrist and be given a series of shock treatments; she may visit a general practitioner and be treated with tranquilizers; she may turn to a minister for spiritual help, to an analyst for psychotherapy, to a friend for a sexual affair, or to an attorney for a divorce.

If we approach this young woman's problem from a medical-psychiatric point of view, we shall assume that she is sick. Accordingly, we must ascertain the nature and seriousness of her illness. If it is a serious, "psychotic" depression, she should be treated with electroshock; if it is a "psychogenic" depression, psychoanalysis may be indicated; whereas, if it is only a reaction to a "mild" or "transient" problem, treatment by the general practitioner or the minister may be acceptable. Though this sort of conceptualization may appear attractive and useful, it is misleading and worthless. Criteria external to the patient's experiences and life style should not lead the therapist to decide whether a particular person with problems in living should be "treated" by psychotherapy, religious counseling, electroshock, or by means of other acts not formally "therapeutic" (e.g., divorce, change of occupation, etc.).

To be sure, a person may seek one type of solution for his problems rather than another because of lack of knowledge of the full range of possibilities available to him. But this argument misses the point; ignorance of this sort is an integral part of the individual's personality or self.

DIAGNOSIS OR DIALOGUE?

Once more, the similarities between the problem of the patient seeking help for difficulties in living and the problem of the student, especially one faced with a career choice, are illuminating. One young man may go into his father's business; another may study music; a third may become a scientist; a fourth, a bricklayer. Each makes a choice, for better or for worse. It is thus possible that the student who drops out of high school and works diligently in an enterprise that is meaningful to him may, in his mature years, conclude that he had acted wisely in his youth; whereas another young man who stays in school and goes on to college and graduate school may experience a serious identity crisis in his forties, when he realizes that he should never have become, say, a lawyer. There is no "objective" way of judging the merit of such occupational choices.

These considerations support the autonomous psychotherapist's attitude toward his client. His conduct must help, not hinder, the patient to make an informed choice in regard to the therapy (if any) he should seek for his problems in living. The therapist can do this by keeping in mind that his task is, first, *not to diagnose the patient, but to engage him in a meaningful dialogue* and, second, not to try to collect data *from* the patient, but to relay appropriate information *to* him.

Frequently, the therapist seeks to gather quickly as much information as possible about the patient. The young social worker is taught to conduct careful and systematic "intake interviews"; the young psychologist, to administer batteries of "diagnostic tests"; and the young psychiatrist, to carry out "diagnostic interviews" to assess the patient's "psychodynamics." All too often, analysts have followed the same strategy; but for them it is a trap. What is the point of this information? Clearly, the physician, the psychologist, the social worker, and so forth need these data because they are expected to render a *decision* —clothed in the mantle of a psychopathological diagnosis. For example, a hospital psychiatrist may refer a patient to a psychologist, expecting the latter to decide, on the basis of certain projective tests, whether the patient suffers from "schizophrenia" or "hysteria." Each of these diagnoses implies certain actions. In sum, an expert needs certain information if he wishes to arrive at a rational judgment and thus decide on a course of action. This is as it should be. But is this the position of the psychoanalyst confronted by a patient seeking analysis?

In most instances, the analyst's clients are preselected, for they are chosen, by themselves or others, as persons desiring or needing analysis. Nevertheless, the problem of patient selection is often discussed as though a therapist and a large, heterogeneous group of "mentally ill" people confronted each other. How they come together is rarely specified. In this view, the analyst's first task is to divide the group into two classes: those who can be analyzed and those who cannot. In reality, this is not the analyst's task. To be sure, there may be a few persons consulting him who know neither what the analyst does nor what they themselves want. But they present no serious problem to the specialist in psychoanalysis.

We must assume that the analyst practices only analysis. (If he uses other methods of a radically different character as well, selection of patients will be difficult for him. I shall not be concerned here with this problem.) Thus, the therapist who offers the patient only a certain type of "help" must explain this to patients who do not already know it. So informed, most patients who want nonanalytic help will promptly leave. Hence, the so-called problem of patient-selection really begins only after the analyst meets a client who understands what he is selling and who wants to purchase it. This situation is fully comparable to that of a well-informed client seeking to purchase the services of an expert.

Ideally, persons who wish to increase their knowledge or improve their skills select themselves for the roles of student or trainee. This is usually the case of the student who applies for admission to a medical school, a law school, or a school of engineering and of the client who seeks the services of a piano teacher or a tennis coach. The patient who seeks the services of an analyst is in a similar position. He is an autonomous agent who selects himself for the role of analysand because he wishes to undergo a process of analytic learning. It is presumptuous for anyone to challenge this right of self-selection. The applicant— especially if he himself pays the expert's fee or the school's tuition—is entitled to choose what he wants to study and, therefore, what he wants to become. Thus, the initial responsibility of the expert, the school, or the psychoanalyst is to provide information so that the client or student can make an informed choice.

In the office practice of psychotherapy today, especially in large cities, the initial selector is usually the client, not the therapist. If the analyst is known for the kind of work he does, many patients will come to him because they want to purchase the kind of service he sells. Had they desired organic treatment or hospitalization, they would have sought psychiatrists known to dispense these commodities.

The Initial Contact between Patient and Autonomous Therapist

In the initial situation in autonomous psychotherapy, there are two persons: a client seeking help and an expert offering his services. The aim of both is to increase the client's choices in the conduct of his life. If the analyst follows the traditional path of the medical therapist, he places the patient in a paradoxical situation. The patient is supposed to learn how to improve his skill in making decisions, but to do this he is deprived of the opportunity to decide whether he wants to become this sort of student (analysand). This will be true whenever the teacher (analyst) arrogates to himself the task of selecting the client for the student role. On the other hand, if the decision rests with the patient, it is he, not the analyst, who must possess the relevant information.

Insofar as the initial interviews serve the purpose of data-collection, information must be gathered, not only by and for the analyst, but also by and for the patient. The initial clarification of the analytic game and the subsequent trial period help the patient understand what analysis entails. Thus informed, he can decide rationally and responsibly whether to undertake analysis.

Thus far, I have emphasized that it is not the therapist but the patient who decides what he will do. This contrasts with the traditional medical relationship, in which the expert decides *for* the client. In autonomous psychotherapy, the client makes all decisions that affect his own life primarily. Not only is he free to decide, but he *must* decide whether he wants to be analyzed and, if he does, by whom. This does not mean, of course, that the patient decides *for* the therapist. Like the patient, the therapist is free to determine—indeed, *must* determine—whether he wishes to lease his services to a particular client who consults him. Though this may seem obvious, its implications are significant.

Let me repeat, the analyst decides about his own conduct. To be sure, this will affect the patient. Nevertheless, the analyst does not judge whether the patient is analyzable, but only whether he himself wishes to serve as the patient's therapist.

To make this decision, the therapist need not make a diagnosis. Since he neither accepts nor rejects the patient on the basis of a diagnosis, why make one? A patient may be considered hysterical, depressed, compulsive, or schizophrenic. All this makes no difference to the autonomous therapist in forming his decision to accept or reject the patient. Even the patient's history, although important for the therapy, is largely irrelevant to this. Actually, the therapist's judgment to accept or reject a patient for analysis rests—and should rest—on such things as the patient's interest in being analyzed, his capacity to be self-observing and self-reflective, his readiness to comply with the rules of analysis, and his ability to pay for the analyst's services. A patient may be analyzable (according to my criteria) and be diagnosed by psychopathologists as anything from normal to schizophrenic. Indeed, even so-called psychopathic personalities may engage successfully in autonomous psychotherapy if no concession is made to them in negotiating the terms of the trial period and the contract.

In sum, only if both client and therapist are free to decide what they wish and are willing to do can they negotiate the conditions for therapeutic collaboration. This informed negotiation is the basis of the analytic contract.

6

The Trial Period

Psychoanalysis as a Game: The Chess Model

Early in the history of psychoanalysis, Freud likened analytic treatment to a game of chess.* He used this analogy not, however, to call attention to the contractual character of the therapeutic relationship, but to some other aspects. For example, he asserted that the analyst who wishes to teach a nonanalytic physician to practice analysis is in a position comparable to that of the chess expert who tries to teach a novice to play chess. In both cases, Freud argued, one can specify only the beginning and end moves in the game; one cannot make general (theoretical) statements about the moves that characterize the middle game; these must be learned by practice.

Freud also used the chess analogy to say some things about the relations between the players. Although the two players cooperate in playing chess, their relation to each other *in* the game is antagonistic. Similarly, although analyst and analysand cooperate in maintaining the analytic situation, their relation to

* "Papers on Technique" [1911–1915], *The Standard Edition of the Complete Psychological Works of Sigmund Freud,* XII (London: Hogarth Press, 1958), 83–173.

each other is, according to Freud, antagonistic. It is so because the patient represses ideas and feelings that the analyst tries to uncover; the patient "resists" the therapist's interpretive efforts; and so forth. Although suggestive, these ideas fall short of the mark.

Except for passing references to the chess analogy in the sense used by Freud, psychoanalytic theoreticians have made no further use of the game as a model of the therapeutic encounter. In an essay written approximately a decade ago, I used the idea of games to emphasize the contractual nature of the psychoanalytic enterprise.° My main point was that, as persons who play a game pledge to obey its rules, so analyst and analysand pledge to follow the rules of the analytic game. Unlike ordinary medical treatment, psychoanalysis is regulated by contract rules, not by status rules.†

Traditional analytic technique has recently been discussed in terms of Stephen Potter's rules of gamesmanship. According to the author, Jay Haley, the analytic game is characterized by a series of devious gambits by the analyst, aimed at putting the patient one down; the patient, in turn, must learn that, no matter what he does, he remains one down; when he is smart enough to realize this, the therapy is concluded.‡ Regrettably, Haley's satirical theory of psychoanalysis is corroborated by certain modern writings on analytic technique. But Haley's account is lopsided; his whole case rests on an exaggeration of the authoritarian, coercive aspects of psychoanalysis; at the same time, its egalitarian, contractual, noncoercive aspects are completely neglected.

To see Haley's satire in proper perspective, we must draw a parallel between psychoanalysis and politics. In the past two centuries, a metamorphosis has occurred in many societies; formerly autocratic governments—so-called closed societies—

° "On the Theory of Psychoanalytic Treatment," *International Journal of Psychoanalysis*, 38 (1957), 166–182.

† See Chapter 7.

‡ *Strategies of Psychotherapy* (New York: Grune & Stratton, 1963), especially Chapter 4 and the Epilogue.

have become more democratic and open. This does not mean that any contemporary society is completely open or free. Just as the United States inherits the Negro problems from its past, so does psychoanalysis inherit many problems from its medical history. A few social defects in a relatively open society do not make it a closed society, nor do a few heteronomous rules make psychoanalysis a purely coercive game of one-upmanship. To be sure, these defects are undesirable and, if left uncorrected, may well destroy the society or the therapy. Our aim should be, therefore, to correct the defects. Freud created a unique "instrument" for exploring the human condition and for enlarging personal freedom. What he created was not perfect; it is for us to improve it.

What Sort of Game Is the Trial Period?

As I have emphasized, the psychoanalytic relationship is not one situation, but many. Viewing this relationship as a game, we will benefit by distinguishing two parts of it—the trial period and the contractual phase.

The trial period is necessary because patient and analyst hardly know each other, but nevertheless seek some sort of partnership. Neither knows the terms on which the other is willing to settle. The trial period is a kind of bargaining situation. Like all bargaining situations, it is a game of strategy of the mixed-motive type; the players have some interests in common, some in opposition. At this point in therapy, patient and therapist are neither partners in a common enterprise nor opponents in a conflict; rather, they are members of a *precarious partnership.* The fate of this partnership is unknown, indeed, cannot be known. In practice, it depends on the specific moves and counter-moves of both participants. Some examples may clarify these comments.*

The client would like to be accepted as a patient by the

* See in this connection also the discussion of the practice of autonomous psychotherapy, especially chapters 10 and 11.

analyst, but he cannot know the analyst's terms until he himself makes some moves. For example, to get what he wants from the analyst, the patient may not know what course to follow. Should he dramatize his symptoms to prove that he is "sick" and thus stimulate the therapist's moral obligation to help him? Should he flatter the analyst to convince him that he is the only therapist who could possibly help him? Or should he drop hints to assure the analyst that money is no consideration and so stimulate the therapist's pecuniary interest in his case?

Conversely, the analyst would like to have an analytic patient —to practice his profession and thus earn a living. But he does not know whether the patient can pay his fee; whether he is willing to pay it; or whether the patient wants advice, reassurance, tranquilizers, or drugs to help him sleep, rather than analysis.

In sum, the partnership between client and analyst is precarious for both. Indeed, it ought to be so; only then is it a genuine bargaining situation. At any time, each may lose the other. Actually, I think that the threat of loss is often greater for the therapist than for the patient, but the patient does not know this. The patient may demand, for example, that the therapist intervene with his wife. The analyst may reject this demand, but not terminate the relationship. But, until the patient has put the analyst to this test, he cannot know this. The analyst, on the other hand, must be prepared to be unyielding on certain matters; if he is not, he forfeits his opportunity to perform his task as an analyst. The question is: How can he stand firm without feeling excessively threatened by the possible loss of the patient? At the same time, the therapist must guard against committing the opposite error; he must not be too demanding. The question is: How can he stand firm and negotiate meaningfully without asking too much from the patient?

First, the analyst will be able to do this only if his terms are minimal. By this I mean that the therapist asks the patient to do or to refrain from doing only those things that are indispensable for preserving the integrity of the analytic game. Whether these terms will seem minimal to the patient depends on his personality, just as whether the fee will seem high or low depends on his financial condition.

Second, the analyst, like the patient, will not be able to play the analytic game unless he can bargain from a position of some strength. By this I mean that he must not be too desperate for money or patients; if he is, he is likely to compromise and meet some of the patient's demands even though this may vitiate the conditions necessary for analysis. It is my impression that therapists, especially young ones, often ruin the analytic game in this way. Usually they do not admit this (or are unaware of it) and complain that they are forced to practice supportive psychotherapy because none of their patients are analyzable. I am often told this by young colleagues, both as their friend and as their analyst. When I inquire into the circumstances of their initial contact with the patient, time and again I discover that they have complied with some of the patient's initial requests (which they might have been able to reject without alienating the patient) and that they then find it impossible to regain their ground.

Third, only if the analyst values autonomy and understands the analytic game will he be able to bargain effectively, and by this I do not mean for a high fee, but for the integrity of the analytic situation and for his own as well as his patient's autonomy. If he does, then—physician or not, with or without formal analytic training—he may with practice become a skilled practitioner of autonomous psychotherapy.

The thesis that one cannot bargain effectively from a position of weakness applies equally to the patient. When a person has lost the power to help himself, when he believes that he has nothing to offer another, in brief, when he is very helpless, then someone else must assume responsibility for him. If no one else does, he will perish.

However, a person who is really so helpless, that is, whose helplessness is not at least partly strategic in character, will never arrive at the analyst's office; he will be eliminated from the game by the analyst's method of making appointments.* At a minimum, the analyst's patient will be sufficiently self-reliant to make his own appointment and to keep it. Even if he then confronts the therapist with nearly complete helplessness, the analyst can still conduct himself autonomously; his move is to indicate to the patient that he sells a certain kind of service and that the nature of this service is not influenced by the patient's desperate need or helplessness. This attitude may seem hard-hearted. I do not believe so; it is merely honest. The patient's plight, however awful, does not obligate the therapist, qua analyst, to help him.†

Confronted with this initial move, the patient will have a choice between seeking another therapist who might respond differently to helplessness and assuming more responsibility for himself. (For some patients, the therapist's initial firm stand may constitute the decisive moment in the therapeutic encounter.) If the patient prefers to leave, he must be free to do so and ought not to be "seduced" into therapy by the analyst. If the patient chooses to stay, the bargaining between him and the therapist continues.

CONFLICT AND COOPERATION IN HELPING SITUATIONS

Let us compare this bargaining model of the trial period of analytic therapy to the traditional medical and the classic Freudian views of it. As ordinary medical thinking has it, the relation between patient and doctor or between analysand and analyst is a simple game of pure cooperation: the patient is sick and wants to get well; the physician is a skilled professional who wants to

* See Chapter 10.
† This is a personal judgment. Those who believe that the patient's plight does obligate the therapist to help him will neither care for autonomous psychotherapy nor wish to practice it. I firmly believe that the therapist is and ought to be a human being first and an analyst second. In many human situations—in and out of his office—the therapist will and ought to be helpful to his fellow man. But I urge that he, as well as those he intends to serve as analyst, keep clearly in mind when the therapist functions as analyst and when he does not.

restore the patient to health. Thus, all the interests of patient and doctor coincide; none conflict.

That great cynic George Bernard Shaw devoted much of his life to exposing such hypocritical accounts of human cooperation. In *The Doctor's Dilemma,* he recast the medical game from pure cooperation into pure antagonism. As Shaw would have it, only the patient is interested in recovering his health. The doctor could not care less about that. He is interested in money; social position; disease as a challenging but abstract problem; the patient as an instructive corpse; and, in the play, in the patient's wife as a sexual object. Though the notion that doctor and patient participate in a harmonious partnership and share identical goals is pure fiction, the Shavian counterimage of complete antagonism is wild exaggeration. If it were true, the medical business would be long defunct.

Like Shaw, Freud was more impressed by the antagonistic elements in the analytic (medical) game than by the cooperative elements; thus his analogy between chess and psychoanalysis. We may also recall that Freud overemphasized the patient's "resistances" to being analyzed; at times he gives the impression that only the analyst is interested in the patient being analyzed, and the patient only in *not* being analyzed. At other times, he likens the analyst to a ferocious lion who "springs once and once only" at the presumably helpless lamb-patient.* What Freud meant was that the analyst must keep his promises, including his promise (threat) to terminate the therapy.

On the whole, I believe that Freud's exaggerated emphasis on the antagonistic elements in the doctor–patient relationship was necessary and salutary; it was an antidote to the deceitful hypocrisy, not only in sexual relationships but in so much else in social life, that Freud opposed. Like Shaw, Freud was a social critic. It is the occupational hazard of the social critic to exaggerate conflict at the expense of cooperation. But let us remember that

* "Analysis Terminable and Interminable" [1937], *Collected Papers* (New York: Basic Books, 1959), V, 316–357.

his purpose is not to stimulate conflict, but on the contrary to encourage more authentic cooperation among men.

The point of all this, for us as students of man, is that both pictures of medicine and of psychoanalysis are partly true; both must be recognized in an adequate game-theoretical analysis of the problem. In other words, psychoanalysis is a complex mixed-motive game combining elements typical of two kinds of game: those of common interest and those of conflict. The psychological dilemma that such human encounters pose is expressed strikingly by an aphorism coined by the great Hungarian writer, Frigyes Karinthy. Commenting on the sad state of affairs between the sexes, that is, between persons who, significantly, are called "lovers," he suggested that the reason for it was that each wanted something different: man, woman, and woman, man.

The relation between analyst and analysand, especially during the trial period, is not unlike the perennial problem between the sexes. The patient wants an analysis; he wants to be an authentic, autonomous, liberated individual, but would like to achieve this as cheaply—psychologically and financially—as possible. To help the patient achieve this goal ought to be one of the analyst's goals, too. But, obviously, it is bound to be one of his subsidiary goals. He is likely to have more personal and pressing desires than helping his patient. In particular, as analyst, the therapist wants an opportunity to exercise his talents in his chosen profession; he would like to be able to perform as an analyst, and for this he needs a suitable analysand. In addition, the therapist wants money and would like to earn it with integrity in the authentic pursuit of his lifework.

This sort of reframing of the aspirations of analysand and analyst suggests that Karinthy was right; virtually all significant human relations—whether between analyst and analysand, husband and wife, employer and employee—are fraught with the dangers inherent in games that combine, in delicate balance, elements of conflict and cooperation. In all such relations, we are faced with the task of *maintaining* this balance. If we shift toward too much cooperation, we sink into uncreative boredom and mediocrity; if we shift toward too much conflict, we risk losing our objects and games.

When Does the Trial Period End?

From the beginning of therapy, the patient will be aware that the therapist is negotiating a certain kind of contract. However, its specifications and implications will not become fully explicit until the contractual phase of therapy. The analyst should not terminate the trial period and begin the contractual phase until the patient knows what the therapist is selling and the therapist is confident that the patient is satisfied with buying only that product. If this requirement is not met, the patient is likely to precipitate situations that will make it difficult for the therapist to adhere to his terms in the contract; the therapist will then be forced either to break the contract (often referred to as "modifying" one's technique) or to terminate the therapy.

Assuming that the trial period has been conducted properly and that the patient is interested in pursuing the task of self-exploration, the stage is set for defining the contract, that is, for settling down to the analytic enterprise. For the analyst, this means, first, that he has accepted the client as his analysand; second, that he will see the patient at regularly scheduled appointments, unless cancellation is unavoidable; and, third, that he will serve as the patient's analyst as long as the patient feels the need for this type of help.

Implicitly, of course, the analyst also promises to do his best as a therapist: he will help the patient clarify his history, his present situation, and his aspirations; he will analyze his verbal and nonverbal productions, his dreams, his "symptoms," his "neurosis," and, last but not least, his transferences.

In sum, the analytic contract obliges the analyst to render certain services to the patient; however, it obliges the analyst to do *only* what he has promised, namely, to analyze. The analytic contract thus differs radically from the usual physician–patient relationship; the latter is not governed by a mutually accepted contract, but rather by the so-called medical or psychological needs of the patient and by the traditional therapeutic obligations of the physician.

In assuming the contract, the analysand obliges himself to do one thing only: to pay the analyst's fee (and to pay it in accordance with the agreed terms). Though there is a tacit understanding between analyst and analysand that the client is buying the analyst's services for a particular purpose (that is, to be analyzed), the analysand must be free to decide how he wants to use the analyst's help. This can be assured only if he is required to comply with only one rule: that he pay the fee. Thus, the patient is entitled to resist the analyst's efforts (however subtle) to change his personality. In no other way can we bring about the condition of authentic self-transformation. Any other requirement will subject the patient to the therapist's heteronomous influence and reward him for coerced, inauthentic personality change.

This arrangement is consistent with the commercial character of the analytic enterprise; the analyst sells something, and the patient buys it. Like any buyer, what the analysand does with his purchase is his business. The analyst cannot say to the patient: "If you are going to use analysis in such and such a way, then I will have to modify the terms of our agreement." Still less can he say, "If you wish to use analysis in a certain way, I will not analyze you," and then terminate the treatment. (In some cases, the analyst may come to such a conclusion, but he ought to do so during the trial period. Once that is over, he must renounce this move in the game.)

I believe that this arrangement is necessary if the patient is to feel, as he should, that the therapy is *his* to do with as he pleases. This was Freud's fundamental ethical idea about psychoanalysis; it was intended as a method of freeing people to live their lives as they saw fit, rather than as their families, their society, or their therapist saw fit. This goal cannot be achieved if the therapist merely enunciates it, but then treats it as an unattainable ideal.

His conduct will reveal whether he believes in it. If he does, he will influence the patient only toward autonomy and freedom, so that he will be able to engage in conduct he wishes to practice and refrain from conduct he wishes to avoid. If he does not, he will influence the patient toward particular types of conduct (e.g., the homosexual toward heterosexuality, the kleptomaniac toward not stealing, the phobic toward braving the phobic situation, and so forth). Though such efforts to combat "symptoms" may be "therapeutically legitimate," they have no place in psychoanalysis. Freud recognized this, yet denied it in the therapeutic technique he advocated for the phobic and obsessional patient.*

* "Lines of Advance in Psycho-Analytic Therapy" [1919], *The Standard Edition of the Complete Psychological Works of Sigmund Freud*, XVII (London: Hogarth Press, 1955), 165–166.

7

The Contractual Phase:

I. The Concepts of

Contract and Status

BEFORE CONSIDERING THE NATURE of the analytic contract, let us examine the nature of contracts generally. This will clarify the difference between my use of the term and that of other psychoanalysts.

WHAT IS A CONTRACT?

In everyday language, the word "contract" designates an agreement between two or more persons to do or refrain from doing something. A contract is a bargain, a compact, or a covenant. The human situation denoted by these nouns—and the acts which bring it about, described by such verbs as "to bargain" and "to contract"—are especially relevant to the law. In legal theory, "contract" is defined as a promise or set of promises protected from breach by law. Thus, the legal definition of contract recognizes that contracts may be broken.

Beginning with Freud, psychoanalysts have treated the agreement between analyst and analysand as though it were a contract. However, they have used the term loosely to refer to any kind of agreement or understanding between client and therapist about what each will and will not do. Nowhere in the literature on psychotherapy have I found a discussion of the specific promises which patient and therapist make to each other nor of the penalties incurred for breaking them. As in my previous writings on psychoanalytic treatment, I shall continue to use the term "contract" in its more narrow sense. What, then, do I mean by analytic contract?

The analytic contract is similar to ordinary (legally binding) contracts between buyers and sellers. Examples of this are the agreements between a person who buys a life insurance policy and the company that underwrites the risk; between the man who purchases real estate or stocks and bonds and the seller; and between the individual who agrees to buy such a service as instruction in dancing or skating and the person who promises to perform the service.

Further, the analytic contract, like the legal contract, seeks clarity rather than vagueness and specifies the remedies available should one of the contracting parties fail to keep his promises. They also differ, however, for ordinary contracts are written, whereas analytic contracts are verbal; also, the participants understand that neither legal nor even social sanctions are available for punishing the party who breaks the contract.

Until now, the analytic game has been defined, at best, in a fragmentary way. It has not specified the moves a player may make if his partner fails to keep his promises. But the penalties for rule-breaking are an integral part of any game; without them, no game can be adequately defined. My account of the analytic game and particularly of the contract will thus include precise specifications, not only of the mutual promises between analyst and analysand, but also statements about the action one partner may take should the other cheat, make a mistake, or prove unfit to play the game.

The Organization of Social Relations

There are two basic principles that regulate human relations—status and contract. Relations governed by status are simpler—legally, psychologically, and socially—than those governed by contract. This view was first developed more than a century ago by Sir Henry Maine in his classic study of ancient law. He noted that, in modern societies, there is a "gradual dissolution of family dependency and the growth of individual obligation in its place" and concluded that "the movement of progressive societies has hitherto been a movement from Status to Contract."[*] We shall first examine these concepts and then use them for clarifying the relationship between physician and patient, psychotherapist and client.

Status and the Family

The family is our most important status relationship. As children, we occupy the statuses (or roles) of son, brother, grandson, and so forth. As adults, if we form families of our own, we establish a complementary set of status relationships. In view of the significance which psychoanalysis and other theories of personality attribute to childhood experiences, the importance for human life of status relationships is evident. To put it differently: as game-players, we begin life by being taught and by learning the rules of status games. It could not be otherwise; because of biological and psychological limitations, small children cannot play contract games.

The model of the family and the status rules which regulate the relations in it are easily extended to larger social groups and to the political community. Primitive society is a large family governed by status obligations and privileges. Likewise, pre-democratic society is a replica of the autocratic family. At its head is the ruler, who is often regarded as divine or endowed

[*] *Ancient Law* [1861] (London: J. M. Dent & Sons, n.d.), pp. 99–100.

with suprahuman faculties; in various positions below him are his subjects, who are indoctrinated to know their proper places. The relations among persons in such a society are predetermined by the rules of the society; what a person may or may not do is part of (and is what we mean by) his status.

All societies were once governed by these principles. Indeed, it is often asserted that groups—committees, organizations, or even entire societies—conduct themselves in a more "primitive" or less conscientious manner than do individuals. And so it seems. Nevertheless, sooner or later, even societies and nations grow up. Like children, they do this by repudiating status relations and electing to be governed by contracts. We have seen this happen in history and can see it happening today, at home as well as abroad. Let me indicate what I mean.

The American Negro is in revolt because he wants to repudiate, once and for all, his *status;* he demands to be treated as a person, not as a Negro. In other words, he wants to be accepted as a contracting individual—as free to contract as the next man—and not as the occupant of a special, inferior status. (Every type of discrimination—whether according to race, religion, or psychiatric criteria—makes use of status relations; each aims to deprive the victim of his right to contract and to transform him into the occupant of a status.)

Abroad, we witness the seething protest of people recently or still colonized; all demand release from the shackles of colonial status and the right to be self-governing—that is, freely contracting—nations. The appeal of Communist ideology to the masses of these so-called underdeveloped countries should occasion no surprise. To people whose lives have been crammed into the narrow confines of lowly statuses, with all escape barred, the Communist political system offers a measure of real freedom. It liberates them from a social game governed by status rules and substitutes one governed by contractual rules. To be sure, the Communist game does not provide man (the ordinary player) with as many moves (as much political freedom) as citizens of a modern Western democracy enjoy.

Let us not forget, however, that, for hundreds of years, the British and the Americans were governed by contract. Their ideal was an agreement freely entered into by both ruler and ruled— the principle of "the consent of the governed." But the Russians and many other people were still living under the autocratic tyranny of a near-divine monarch or chieftain. No contract was safe against his whim. Indeed, the term "absolute ruler" refers to the head of a state endowed with unrestrained power; he is unfettered by contract. The essence of contract, at least in this context, is *restraint of power*. If a contract is to be meaningful there must be effective provisions for its fulfillment.

Contract and Modern Society

Contract is at once an ancient phenomenon and a relatively modern one. The ancient Hebrews made a covenant with Jehovah; they promised specific religious observances in return for God's promise to treat them as his chosen people. On a more informal scale, the Greeks and Romans made bargains—a species of contract—with their gods. And, of course, these ancient people made binding agreements among themselves.

All this is to be expected. For to make and break promises is an exquisitely human faculty. Nietzsche, who so strongly influenced Freud, even suggested that "to breed an animal that is able to make promises . . . is the task which Nature set for herself."* The result is man. So far as we know, no other animal has this capability. Although Nietzsche's insight was brilliant, we must see it in context. The fact that man makes promises is a consequence of his other unique abilities, namely, to make and use signs, to construct rules and languages, and to organize games. Thus, to play a language game, which is a basic human capacity, is to engage in an exercise involving obligations and promises; the speakers pledge to use mutually accepted signs and sign-rules. (It is hardly surprising, therefore, that we regard the schizophrenic, who breaks this promise, as infrahuman.)

* Quoted by Harold C. Havighurst, *The Nature of Private Contract* (Evanston, Ill.: Northwestern University Press, 1961), p. 12.

Although a fundamental human quality, ancient in its roots, contracting has only recently achieved social significance in everyday life. Perhaps this is because a contract is, by and large, an arrangement between equals; it rejects coercion and fosters freedom. Though present in some form in the ancient or primitive worlds, these ideas and phenomena have flourished only in the West, and only since the Renaissance. In earlier times, social arrangements were based on relations among unequals—between strong and weak, freeman and slave, ruler and subject. Such relations were coercive, grounded on command, rather than cooperative, based on contract; they fostered group solidarity and social rigidity, rather than individualism and social fluidity.

In all contemporary societies, the significance of status relations is diminishing while that of contractual relations is increasing. There are several reasons for this. A process of social leveling, active in both the democracies and the Communist nations, is eradicating the vast inequities of social class and wealth typical of preindustrial, feudal societies. The influence of family and church, the two institutions regulated by status rather than by contract, is steadily diminishing. At the same time, the individual, as a unit of social structure, is gaining importance—despite arguments about "mass man" and "organization man." As a result, the necessity and significance of contract as a method of regulating social relations are rapidly increasing.

Actually, when dignified individuals wish to engage in an enterprise requiring the efforts of more than one man, there is but one method for creating cooperation among them—the contract. The difference between contract and command becomes ever sharper. The former appeals to incentives; the latter, to punishments. The man who commands threatens to harm his fellow man; the one who contracts promises to help him. Command is sadomasochistic; contract, mutually hedonistic. And, perhaps most important for our interest in autonomous psychotherapy, command implies slavery, whereas contract implies freedom. The person who is commanded may choose between obeying and being punished; the person offered a contract, among accepting the contract, rejecting it, or continuing to negotiate.

Contracts and promises thus tend to enlarge the range of independent action; commands and statuses, to narrow it. Students of contract have gone so far as to assert that "contract *is* freedom."* Actually, the two concepts are so intertwined that we may also state that freedom is freedom *to* contract. Finally, contract enhances the moral posture of man by limiting the opportunities for a man to injure another. The opportunity to maim, rob, and kill, as Justice Holmes said, "is open to the whole world of the unscrupulous."† The law may punish the villain, but that is scant help to the victim. Contract limits the opportunity for being injured to those with whom one has chosen to deal. Although there are vast numbers of persons willing to break contracts, we are free *not* to make contracts with them. Thus, by judicious selection, a man can limit the circle of those who can hurt him by failing to keep a promise.

As I suggested earlier, contracts are strategies in the service of an enlightened hedonism; they seek to maximize pleasures and to minimize pains. Thus, contracts regulating relations extending over long periods must foresee and provide for future contingencies. Many contracts do this. Controversies between the contracting parties may thus be settled before they arise. The analytic contract must also do this; analyst and analysand must anticipate possible difficulties and prepare the solution in advance, for example, what to expect if one or the other cancels an appointment, goes on vacation, and so forth.

Status, Contract, and the Physician–Patient Relationship

The actual relations between physicians and patients are complex. Some are regulated by status rules; others, by contracts; and the majority, by a combination of the two methods. What

* *Ibid.*, p. 35.
† *Ibid.*, p. 69.

produces these various medical situations? In general, the pattern adopted depends on the social positions of the participants. In a two-person (or two-group) interaction, if one of the parties is more sophisticated and socially more powerful, he will tend to dominate the other. If, however, both parties are equal or nearly so, they are likely to adopt a contractual, mutually cooperative relationship. Thus, not only may physicians dominate patients, but patients, physicians.

If the patient is poor or feels helpless because of his illness, the physician may exploit the situation by assuming a superior position; he may command the patient to submit to his edicts or suffer the consequences. Penalties for trying to repudiate the inferior role of patient vary. The patient may lose the services of the physician or be subjected to diagnostic or therapeutic procedures medically rationalized and justified but unnecessary and painful. (As a young physician, I often saw doctors perform unnecessary spinal punctures on uncooperative patients—charity cases, of course.) Or the person may be punished by legal or social sanctions, for example, by commitment to a mental hospital.

However, if the patient is more powerful, the physician may be placed in an inferior position. This happens less often than the reverse, but is by no means unknown. In societies where vast social and economic inequalities prevail, the physician is apt to be relatively poor and socially unimportant. Thus, he may find himself at the mercy of wealthy and politically powerful persons or families. The patient will then command, and the physician obey. Attempts by the physician to repudiate his lowly status may be punished by sanctions ranging from economic hardship to loss of life. The physician who becomes the agent of a powerful institution is like his colleague, the captive employee of a powerful family in a feudal system; he abandons his independence which is rooted in equality with a multiplicity of individual clients who are also his sources of income.

These are some of the economic and political attributes of the physician–patient relationship that may cause it to be unbalanced. It may also be unbalanced for medical and psychological reasons.

The medical situation—of which the analytic situation has traditionally been considered a subspecies—is usually a replica of the family situation. As the parent cares for the child, so the doctor cares for the patient. The role of physician and analyst as a healer and as a responsible, parentlike figure is thoroughly entrenched in psychoanalytic thinking. (Some psychoanalysts firmly believe that "fatherly" and "motherly" persons are especially effective analysts.) This conception of the analytic situation has far-reaching implications.

If the relationship between analyst and patient is like that between father and child, then, by definition, it is inimical to the aim of analysis. How can the analyst help his client become autonomous and free in the conduct of his own life if the relationship between them is based on status, with the patient cast in the inferior rank, and, further, if the analyst subjects the patient to a heteronomous influence, based on authority and command?

The faulty analogy of analyst and parent or of analyst and medical healer is misleading in another respect. This traditionally "therapeutic" posture implies a virtually limitless devotion by the analyst to the analysand. Many physicians and psychotherapists cultivate this attitude. Thus, the so-called supportive psychotherapist, believing that his very "caring" for the patient is itself therapeutic, fosters the patient's credulity about the therapist's involvement with him. The existential therapists, too, if one may judge by a recent exposition of their work,* encourage the idea that the therapist must have a limitless dedication to his patient's welfare. If the patient becomes psychotic, the therapist cares for him; if he cannot feed himself, the therapist feeds him; and so forth.

This posture is a sham. Like the parent or the physician, the therapist, too, has his limits beyond which he cannot or will not care for his patient. Pledged to be absolutely honest with the patient, the analyst must recognize his limits and inform the patient of them. If he were to act otherwise, he would be making

---

* Medard Boss, *Psychoanalysis and Daseinsanalysis,* trans. Ludwig B. Lefebre (New York: Basic Books, 1963).

promises he could not keep. No person and certainly no psychotherapist can pledge to take complete care of another. Should
the patient become psychotic, require hospitalization and constant attention like a sick infant, how could the therapist fulfill
his promise of unlimited care to this patient without breaking
his promise to another? And how could he keep his promises to
others—his wife, children, and friends? The therapist who creates
the impression that his devotion and duty to the patient are
boundless is an impostor, for the aim of this strategy is to
aggrandize himself and render his patients dependent, grateful,
and guilty.

Freud realized that the analytic situation differs significantly
from the medical situation. Accordingly, he scrutinized the medical situation and adapted it to the requirements of analysis. But,
in my opinion, he only made a beginning. The analytic game he
constructed and which his followers institutionalized suffers from
many inadequacies. In particular, it retains too many of the status
aspects of the medical game. By the same token, it is not sufficiently contractual. My aim has been to continue the work that
Freud began and to transform psychoanalysis into a *fully* contractual type of psychotherapy. What is meant by this will, I
hope, become clear in this book.

CONTRACT AS COMMUNICATION

Let us now examine contract as a particular kind of communication. The analyst is principally an expert in decoding the patient's disguised messages. Though important, this function of
the therapist deflected attention from scrutinizing *his* communications with the patient. In the past, the analyst's communications
have been thought of mainly as clarifications, interpretations, and
questions. In other words, the analyst translates from the language of the patient into the language of the analysis. But this
is not all he does.

The analyst also makes promises. Promises or contracts form
a special class of communications. They are not assertions about

facts nor are they clarifications, interpretations, translations, or questions. Promises are statements about the speaker's *future* behavior; they are communications about his intention to follow certain rules. However, not every statement about one's future behavior is a true promise. Herein lies one of the differences between assuming a status role and making a contract.

For example, if a therapist says or implies that he will try to cure a patient's neurosis, this is not a promise. It is not clear what sort of conduct is required of the therapist to keep it or break it. Some would interpret the statement as an obligation to analyze the patient; others, to give him electroshock treatments; still others, to reassure him; and so forth.

Contracts or promises are meaningful in proportion to their exactness. If Peter and Paul agree to meet at the corner of First and Main at 5 o'clock on Tuesday, this is a contract; if they agree to meet after work, it is not. The essence of a promise lies in the *constraint* it places on the promiser's future behavior. By asserting what one's future conduct will be, one relinquishes a measure of freedom about it. The person who says to another, "I shall meet you at 5:00 P.M." is physically free to act otherwise. However, he is morally obligated to keep his promise by acting according to the agreement.

Thus, if autonomous psychotherapy is to be contractual, the therapist cannot make vague promises to the patient, such as "I will take care of you," "I will protect your best interests," or even "I will analyze you." Instead, he must promise to do and avoid doing certain specific things. This is why I emphasize such seemingly unimportant details as the analyst's obligation not to prescribe drugs, communicate with third parties, and so forth. Only in terms of such concrete acts can a meaningful contract be formulated. Moreover, once an adequate contract has been arranged and both parties have agreed to it, it is easy to identify conduct that violates the terms of the agreement. For example, some patients are worried about the analyst's participation in their life. In contemplating suicide, they may want the analyst to save them and also to leave them alone to die; or they may want the analyst to hospitalize them forcibly and also to trust them to be their own masters.

If the analyst merely promises to discharge his obligation as a doctor or psychotherapist, he does not specify the conduct that this will entail. Indeed, he can easily make this kind of promise, for he remains free to act as he chooses. But the essence of a promise is that it curtails the promiser's freedom of action; if it does not, it is not an effective promise. Accordingly, there are many activities from which the analyst must pledge to abstain; making "therapeutic" decisions about hospitalizing the patient or protecting him from commiting suicide (by extra-analytic maneuvers) are two such acts. This is a promise that the analyst can keep and one that is consistent with his other promises to the analysand. Having established this contract, the analyst is no longer free to consider the question, "Should I commit Mr. Jones to prevent his suicide?" He has relinquished his freedom to act in this matter. He *can,* of course, hospitalize Mr. Jones; but he does so at the cost of his moral commitment to the patient. Nor does the matter stop there; the therapist's contract violation is likely to become known and to affect his relations with other patients and colleagues.

FREEDOM TO CONTRACT

Freedom is an essential ingredient of contract. Indeed, it is meaningless to speak of a contract between persons who are not free. This fact is significant for psychiatry and psychoanalysis because psychotherapists frequently form relationships with patients under circumstances in which one or both are not free to contract. As a result, the vast majority of encounters between psychiatrists and patients and even many between analysts and their clients *cannot* be contractual and are therefore not analytic.

For example, the patient may be a child, a prisoner, or a person commited to a mental institution. None of these persons can enter into the sort of two-person contract necessary for analytic work. Nor can the poor person who cannot pay the analyst for his services. Hence, although a person may be "analyzable" (in the traditional sense), analysis may still be impossible. To the prison and the mental hospital, we may add the military services and totalitarian societies; each constitutes a social situation in which the analytic contract cannot be realized because of the limitations placed on one or both parties. In proportion as either therapist or patient is not free—in particular, not free with respect to the conduct of their relationship with each other—there is an external, situational limit on psychoanalysis. This limit is insurmountable regardless of the professional qualifications of the therapist and the psychological make-up of the patient.

The idea is not new that the analysand must be a socially free and independent person. Freud said that he tried to follow the rule "of not taking on a patient for treatment unless he was *sui juris,* not dependent on anyone else in the essential relations of his life."* But, having said it, he and other analysts proceeded to disregard its implication and spoke of the "analysis" of children, prisoners, hospitalized psychotics deprived of all human rights, and so forth. Those who speak this way forget that we cannot use the verb "to analyze" transitively and mean by it psychoanalysis as autonomous psychotherapy. Such usage implies an activity, by a subject on an object, as when a chemist "analyzes" an unknown substance. But nothing like this occurs in psychoanalysis. In this context, "to analyze" means, among other things, to contract with someone; if the therapist's partner is not in a position to contract, it is absurd to speak of analysis.

By the same token, there can be no analysis if the analyst is not in a position to contract. This possibility, though real and frequent, is generally ignored. (Perhaps it is not only neglected, but denied.) When is the analyst not free to contract for an analysis? This happens most often when the therapist is the patient's employer or employee or his superior in a training system that is authoritarian and coercive.

* "Introductory Lectures on Psychoanalysis" [1915–1917], *The Standard Edition of the Complete Psychological Works of Sigmund Freud,* XV–XVI (London: Hogarth Press, 1963), 460.

For example, the analyst may be the chairman of a department of psychiatry, and the patient, his resident or a member of his staff. Conversely, the patient may be a university professor while the analyst may hold a lesser appointment in the medical school. Sometimes the therapist is employed by the university to analyze residents or junior staff members (and is paid partly or wholly by the institution, not by his patients). Or the patient may be professionally prominent or exceptionally wealthy and thus able to benefit the analyst in ways other than by only paying his bills. In each of these cases, there is an actual or potential conflict of interest between the therapist's role as analyst and as beneficiary of the patient's largess or between the patient's role as analysand and as beneficiary of the analyst's largess. Some conflicts of interest of this type can be recognized in advance and prevented. If the integrity of the analytic situation can be preserved (and this may depend partly on the personalities of the two individuals), then an analytic contract can be negotiated and analytic work carried out. However, if conflicts of interest remain unrecognized—or, worse, are ignored and allowed to have an unanalyzed extra-analytic existence—then the analysis will be a sham.

This is the case with contemporary training analysis. The training analyst is not free to contract; his essential liberty toward the analysand is curtailed by the rules and regulations of the psychoanalytic training system. When the interests of the patient and of the educational organization conflict, those of the latter prevail.

The position of the training analyst vis-à-vis the candidate is comparable to that of the state hospital psychiatrist vis-à-vis the committed patient (or vice versa). In the state mental hospital, neither the staff psychiatrist nor the committed patient is free; the psychiatrist is compelled to "take care" of the patient, and the patient is forced to assume the sick role. The two cannot contract, since each is deprived of the freedom to act responsibly toward his partner. Thus, the committed patient is not permitted to hire and fire the psychiatrist, dispose of his funds, regulate his movements in space and time, and so forth. Similarly, the training analyst is not permitted to safeguard the confidences of his candidate-patient, set the fee, allow the patient autonomy in the conduct of his life, and so forth.

There may be still other restrictions on both the candidate's and the training analyst's liberty to contract with each other. The assignment of the training analyst to the candidate and of the candidate to the training analyst; the frequency of the sessions; the minimum length of the analysis; the patient's position on the couch—all these may be determined by third parties. In brief, the contract between training analyst and psychoanalytic institute and the one between candidate and institute leave little room for a contractual relationship between candidate and training analyst. This has been one of the tragic mistakes of psychoanalysis as a profession. It is probably the main reason that the autonomous and contractual features of psychoanalysis have so long remained in embryonic form. Like a fetus deformed by a field of heavy ionizing radiation, psychoanalysis has been deformed by the social field through which its practitioners have had to pass.

The analytic training system is inimical to the basic values of psychoanalytic treatment as autonomous therapy. The early promise of psychoanalysis as contractual psychotherapy has thus come to naught. Instead, we have witnessed the birth and growth of our contemporary psychotherapeutic monster—institutionalized, medicalized psychoanalysis. This "psychoanalysis" is a cohesive professional discipline, an influential social movement, and a powerful ideology. But, as a form of human helpfulness, it is a misfit. It is neither bona fide medical therapy, organic-directive psychiatry, nor Freudian psychoanalysis; instead, it is an unpredictable mixture of all these elements.

8

The Contractual Phase:
II. Contract Bridge and
Contractual Psychotherapy

From Trial Period to Contract

It is useful, both for conceptualizing the therapeutic encounter
and for conducting the analysis, to consider the trial period as
one phase of therapy and the contractual phase as another. At
the same time, it is necessary to have a clear idea about the
connection between these two phases of the treatment.

In terms of game theory, the trial period is a mixed-motive
game, and the contractual period, a common-interest game. During
the trial period, some of the players' aims coincide, whereas
others conflict; during the contractual phase, their interests progressively converge. Though this may be considered an ideal, it
is often possible to approximate it in practice.

What is the connection between the trial phase and the contractual phase? Although I have described them as two different

kinds of game, they are actually two phases of the same game. The trial and contractual phases of autonomous psychotherapy are related functionally; the former is an introductory or preliminary stage which may or may not lead to a subsequent working stage. There is a similar relation between courtship and marriage in the family game; between negotiation and settlement (and working) in the bargaining game; and between bidding and playing a hand in a game of bridge.

In each of these cases, we witness a two-phase sequence of human relations: a period of precarious partnership followed by one of secure partnership. Thus, the marriage game, if played autonomously, presupposes that the participants will try to get to know each other and will coordinate their goals and expectations for their potential union. Unless they have the "same interests" for the marriage—that is, unless they propose to play a common-interest game as husband and wife—the relationship will founder on conflict.

Clearly, then, if we wish to find a game model for the analytic relationship, it ought to be bridge, not chess. Indeed, by analyzing the structure of this game, we gain a useful lever for understanding psychoanalysis.

BRIDGE AND PSYCHOANALYSIS

Bridge is a complex game, partly one of chance and partly one of strategy. Further, though each team engages the other in a game of pure conflict, between themselves the partners play a game of pure coordination. Finally, the game is biphasic; a period of bidding precedes the playing of the hand. However, if we wish to use bridge as a model for psychoanalysis, we must concentrate on those aspects of the game that are important for our purposes. Thus, we shall skip over the dealing of cards and hence the element of chance in the game; we shall also ignore the competitive relationship between the two teams. What remains is two players—the partners of one team—each with thirteen cards in his hand.

A basic similarity between bridge (auction or contract) and contractual psychotherapy is that both are biphasic games; each starts from an initial position characterized by mutual exploration and only tentative commitment to a future collaboration. Each evolves to one of two kinds of later situation. If an agreement can be reached, there will be a contract and hence a mutual commitment to a pure common-interest game; if no agreement can be reached, there will be no contract. In the case of bridge, this may mean that a new hand will be dealt or that the defending team will collaborate, not in playing a hand or fulfilling a contract, but in attempting to defeat their opponents. In the case of patient and therapist, this means that they may part company, or they may decide to continue a tentative relationship without promises of a more permanent contractual commitment. This is like a prolonged engagement which may end in either separation or marriage. Occasionally, patients prefer not to enter into a committed situation of any kind; a prolonged trial period may thus ensue. If adequate mutual autonomy can be maintained, there is no valid reason for the analyst not to accept this sort of provisional arrangement. Indeed, for some patients, most of the therapy may take place in what the analyst might consider the trial phase.

Auction Bridge and Contract Bridge

The differences between auction and contract bridge are more instructive than the similarities. As the terms imply, auction bridge resembles a process of auctioning; contract bridge, a process of contracting. The terms are apt and may be taken quite literally. As in an auction, the bidding in auction bridge tends to be unrestrained, for, to play a hand, each team must outbid the other. Moreover, the penalties for overbidding and not fulfilling one's contract are light. Thus, the game rules of auction bridge encourage enthusiastic bidding in the hope that, with luck, the player will be able to complete his bid. It is significant, finally, that, though it is necessary for the two partners to communicate with each other (for example, to establish which suit to play), the need to do so is not very great. Rather, each player is apt to play selfishly and to be more interested in his own hand and what he can do with it than in establishing a solid partnership with his partner.

Contract bridge, though resembling auction bridge in some of its external trappings—such as the cards used and the rules for playing a hand—is a radically different sort of game. The rules of contract bridge do not place a premium on playing a hand; on the contrary, defending a hand can be more profitable. Hence, the standard of bidding is not that of an auction; the higher, the better. One cannot buy anything at an auction by bidding low, although one may save money that way. Just so, one cannot win at auction bridge by consistently careful and restrained bidding.

In contract bridge, on the other hand, bidding is for each player to inform his partner of the strength and weakness of his own hand so that they may arrive at a contract they can fulfill. In the long run (with evenly matched players), that team will win which neither underbids nor overbids habitually. The team that underbids fails to make the score it could have made; it may also let the opposing team play and score, even though it could have bettered its opponents' bid. The team that overbids is seriously penalized for failing to realize its contract.

Contract Bridge and Contractual Psychotherapy

There is a close parallel between contract bridge and contractual psychotherapy. The bridge-players get acquainted by bidding; patient and therapist get acquainted by engaging in certain moves during the trial period. In both games, each player must try to ascertain what his partner has or wants and must also notify his partner of what he himself has or wants. Initially, the partnership is precarious. Neither participant knows what will come of it; each bases his plans for future action on the information he receives from his partner. Thus, in contract bridge, what one player bids depends on what his partner has bid (and also on what his opponents have bid; but we may disregard this) and also on the cards he holds.

If a person is committed to playing this game and not some other, he will be influenced by his partner's moves, but only within certain limits; he will not himself make a move inconsistent with the cards he holds. In brief, a good bridge-player will not make promises he cannot keep (unless he deliberately bids a contract that he knows he cannot fulfill to frustrate his opponents—another bridge situation that we must disregard).

The trial period preceding the contractual phase of psychoanalysis is comparable to bidding in contract bridge. In each case, the players are interested either in converting a mixed-motive game into a largely cooperative one or in rejecting a mutually binding partnership. In bridge, the partners try to arrive at a contract they can fulfill; if the bidding indicates that this cannot be done, they agree not to contract. Similarly, client and analyst try to settle on a mutually satisfying contract; but, if they cannot, they decide not to enter into a binding therapeutic relationship.

In this type of game situation, the players can attain their goals only by conveying to each other the *truth* about their own behavior and expectations. I emphasized previously that patient and analyst must honestly communicate what each offers the other. If the players are untruthful, they mislead each other and render their later cooperation difficult or impossible. In particular, the therapist who promises—by word or act (for example, through certain moves in the initial phase of therapy)—to do things for the patient that subsequently he does not want to or cannot do acts like the bridge player who overbids his hand; when he shows it to his partner, the latter realizes that he has been deceived. Like bridge players who mislead each other, patients and therapists who act in this fashion suffer joint defeat.

Two Types of Bridge Game—Two Types of Psychotherapy

The differences between auction and contract bridge help explain the differences between loosely organized (chaotic) psychotherapies based on "psychodynamic understanding" and (contractual) psychoanalysis.

Although the differences may seem small or subtle, auction and contract bridge are two radically different games. The similarities pertain to nonessentials, such as the cards and the structure of the game. The inexperienced bridge-player will be impressed by the similarities between auction and contract bridge; the expert, by the differences. Indeed, the latter may see auction bridge as the opposite of contract bridge or as a corrupted version of it. (Actually, auction bridge was devised first; it was later refined into contract bridge.)

Many of the same things could be said and often are said about two types of psychotherapeutic game, namely, so-called psychoanalytically oriented psychotherapy (hereafter also called "psychodynamic therapy" or "rapport therapy") and psychoanalysis. The similarities between them are superficial; the differences, basic. To be sure, both enterprises consist largely of the exchange of verbal and nonverbal communications between a patient and a therapist meeting in a professional setting, usually the therapist's office. However, the two differ radically in the aim of the therapy and the conduct of the participants. Indeed, to the expert in the therapy game, the two may even appear antithetical. Of course, the polarity, often drawn, between rapport therapies and psychoanalysis is a judgment; like all judgments, it reveals something, not only about the object, but also about the individual judging it and his particular interests. To a person who knows little about card games, the similarities between auction bridge and contract bridge will far outweigh the differences, whereas, to a bridge expert, auction bridge is a sacrilege, undeserving of the name "bridge."

The situation is the same in psychotherapy. To the internist or the surgeon or even to the organic psychiatrist, the similarities between psychodynamic therapies and analysis are great, and the differences, insignificant. However, to the psychoanalyst, the social scientist, and to many persons seeking psychotherapy, the differences between rapport therapies and psychoanalysis often are—and certainly ought to be—far more significant than the similarities. Let us review these differences, making use of the contrast between auction and contract bridge.

The Bidding—the Trial Period

Bridge and psychoanalysis are two-phase games. In each, the players have a proximal goal and a distal goal, the former being a means to the latter. In each, the character of the first period of the game—bidding in bridge and the trial period in psychotherapy—will depend on whether bridge is auction or contract and whether psychotherapy is psychodynamic or autonomous.

What is the purpose of the initial phase in each of these games? In auction bridge, defense being a less interesting and rewarding strategy than offense, the partners will aim less at informing each other correctly of the cards they hold than at forming a working partnership. Hence, each player is likely to make "promises" to his partner which he may not be able to keep, by overbidding or otherwise misinforming him.

More specifically, in auction bridge the object of bidding is to name the trump suit or to name "no trump." There is no penalty for underbidding. Regardless of how low the bid, the player and his partner score all the tricks they win; in other words, contracts may be profitably overfulfilled. Furthermore, the penalties for overbidding and underfulfilling one's contract are slight. This makes bidding in auction bridge much less responsible than in contract bridge.

The general practice of psychiatry—especially of nonanalytic, noncontractual psychotherapy—is built on the same principles as auction bridge. The initial period is in the service of a particular goal, namely, that each participant do his utmost to get along with the other so that a "therapeutic relationship" may develop. Thus, patient and therapist do not use this period to inform each other of their mutual expectations. Instead, the therapist overbids his hand by offering the patient whatever he thinks the patient needs or wants; his principal goal is to hold on to the patient long enough to make him interested in "therapy." The patient is likely to play a complementary game; he does his utmost to be a "good patient," to avoid being rejected by the therapist and thus forfeiting his chance to be cured.

Like the players of auction bridge, the therapist and patient who act this way squander the first phase of their encounter. They do not use this opportunity to prepare themselves for a more harmonious future collaboration. On the contrary, they deceive themselves and each other into believing that they ought to worry about only one thing at a time. They behave as though they believed in taking what they can get, in accordance with the maxim, " A bird in hand is worth two in the bush." Thus, the players of auction bridge are satisfied if they can agree on a remotely plausible contract that will permit them to play; they will worry later about fulfilling it.

Similarly, rapport therapist and patient are satisfied if they can establish a remotely plausible therapeutic partnership that will give the therapist a chance to subject the patient to the kind of treatment that the therapist thinks he ought to have and that will give the patient a chance to subject himself to the kind of therapeutic influence that he thinks will help him; they will worry later about the "therapy" being therapeutic or noxious. And worry they will. Under these circumstances, the partnership is ill prepared to function in an honest, workmanlike fashion once it has the chance to do so. Only then do the team-mates discover that they have misinformed each other and that they have not achieved a situation of pure cooperation, but, in fact, one of unclarified conflict. What begins as noncontractual psychotherapy soon becomes chaotic psychotherapy. Neither therapist nor patient knows what the other is up to; instead of collaborating in a joint endeavor, each is busy protecting himself from the intrusions of the other.

In contract bridge, the players try to arrive at a contract they can fulfill. If this seems impossible, they must try to defeat the contract that their opponents made and will attempt to fulfill. Overbidding is severely penalized and is therefore avoided; underbidding is also costly. (A distinctive feature of contract bridge is that a pair cannot score the tricks it wins toward making a game unless it has contracted to win those tricks; in auction bridge, it can.)

Bidding is a far more important part of contract than of auction bridge. It is relatively easy to learn to play one's cards properly; it is more difficult and requires coordination with one's partner to learn to bid well. Genuine expertness in contract bridge lies largely in bidding accurately and yet imaginatively. Each player must come to a precise understanding with his partner about what, as a team, they can and ought to do and also what they cannot and ought not do. If the contract has been correctly negotiated, that is, if the bidding was proper, a competent player can usually fulfill it. The game rules of contract bridge also reward good bidding. Earning the privilege of playing a hand is no advantage at all; the defending team can score as effectively.

The trial period serves the same purpose for psychoanalysis as bidding does for contract bridge. First, therapist and patient must communicate about the sorts of thing they want from and can offer to each other. If they can, they will then arrive at a contract (to play psychoanalysis); but they will not commit themselves to this contract unless they are confident that they can fulfill it. Like bidding in contract bridge, the trial period is set in a context where mere agreement between the players— based on idle hopes and false promises—is discouraged. Both patient and therapist proceed with the understanding that they must first get acquainted; only then will they consider merging into a partnership committed to a definite task. Further, they understand and agree that it is better not to form a partnership than to form one that cannot meet its obligations.

The trial period in contractual psychotherapy is therefore a highly responsible enterprise for both participants. Unlike those embarking on chaotic psychotherapy, the autonomous therapist and his patient maintain a precarious partnership—that is, they prolong the trial period—until it is either dissolved or transformed into a secure partnership. In contrast, the chaotic psychotherapist and his patient usually do not realize how precarious their partnership is until after they have convinced themselves that it was secure.

Playing One's Cards—Fulfilling the Therapeutic Contract

Because of the structure of auction bridge, the players have no incentive to bid accurately or to bid higher than necessary (except to take the play from their opponents). As long as the trump suit is correctly selected, a low bid is as good as a high one for scoring toward the game and, of course, is safer, for it protects against undertricking. Thus, each player will try to play his own hand or help his partner play his; also, each player will try to name trump accurately and to bid as low as possible. As a result, the tricks taken during the play are rarely the number announced in the bid. The game is, therefore, noncontractual or contractual only in a very loose sense.

In contract bridge, one must bid accurately, to the highest score that can be realized, for there is no credit (toward making the game) for unbid tricks. Thus, each player will try to bid informatively and precisely; he will also try either to bid as high as he thinks he can realize (up to game or slam) or to defeat his opponents. As a result, the number of tricks taken during play is often the same as was declared in the final bid. The game is exquisitely contractual.

The conduct of psychodynamic therapies is comparable to

playing one's cards in auction bridge. The partners make only the vaguest sort of agreement: in bridge, they agree only on the suit; in psychotherapy, only on the type of relationship (psychological rather than, say, surgical or dermatologic). But, within these broad limits, what the relationship will be like is not clear in advance. Indeed, the therapist often plans to implement his ideas about the therapy only after the patient has committed himself to the partnership; this is frequently true of the patient as well. Thus, the work phase of therapy readily becomes, not a clear contract, but a chaotic conflict, each participant trying to induce the other to play by *his* rules and to pursue *his* aims.

Faced with this sort of situation, the therapist is likely to resort to constant revision of the relationship and of the "understanding" between him and the patient. For example, the therapist may begin with a confidential two-person relationship, using conversation only. Soon, the patient may become depressed and unable to sleep; the therapist may respond by prescribing drugs —Revision Number One. The depression may deepen, and the therapist may worry that the patient may kill himself; he may now recommend hospitalization and in-patient treatment—Revision Number Two. And so on.

Other changes may serve the therapist's needs more directly. For example, if the therapist wishes to raise his fee, he may reduce the frequency of the patient's appointments and increase the fee; or, if he feels in need of a block of free time, he may give his patient an "interruption"; or, if he tires of a patient, he may terminate his treatment.

The distinctive feature of psychoanalysis is the contract. It limits the therapist in the sorts of thing he can do vis-à-vis the patient. He has a contract with the patient and is honor-bound (for the present, not legally bound) to obey its terms. Nor can the therapist alter the contract because the patient asks him to. On the contrary, such a request is important grist for the analytic mill.

There is one important difference between the analytic contract and the "contract" to which partners in bridge agree, namely, the power of each player vis-à-vis his partner. Partners at bridge are equals; each player can help or harm his partner about as much as the latter can help or harm him. This is not true in the case of psychoanalysis; the analyst can help or harm the patient more than the patient can the analyst. The client is in a weaker position than the therapist. The analytic contract serves in part to reduce this inequality and protect the patient from the analyst's power.

In this respect, we may take the United States Constitution as our model of the analytic contract. It, too, is an agreement between two parties who are morally equal, but in fact (socially) unequal—the governors and the governed. What does it specify? Significantly, it requires little of the governed; implicitly, of course, they are asked to obey the law. Principally, however, the Constitution (and other documents like it) specifies certain things that those in power must do and must avoid doing. In effect, it is a promise by them to limit their own power. In the discharge of governmental duties, they eschew arbitrary authority and discretionary action in favor of specific restraints, for example, due process.

As I conceive it, the analytic contract sets out to do the same thing. In the exercise of the traditional healing function, the therapist renounces arbitrary power and the discretionary judgments by which it is usually justified in favor of specific restraints. Of course, this attitude can be maintained only toward the patient who assumes responsibility for his conduct and its social consequences.

Freedom, Coercion, and the Psychoanalytic Relationship

The traditional analyst lays down certain rules for the patient and justifies them by appealing to the interests of "therapy." This is a deceptive argument, easily misused; we should be wary of it. In actuality, there is no such thing as "therapy"; there is only a particular therapist, a particular patient, and their communications, especially their promises, to each other. In principle, the "needs of analysis" require and justify the idea that therapist and patient follow certain rules. In practice, however, "the therapy" has no needs; only the therapist and the patient do.

It is therefore not enough for the analyst to mouth his commitment to the ethic of autonomy; he must live it. If the ethic of autonomy is fundamental to psychoanalysis, its practice must begin at home, in the analytic situation. This is the most important reason for the analyst not to impose various kinds of rules on the patient, other than the minimal and agreed-upon rules necessary for autonomous psychotherapy.

These considerations converge on a single proposition: to preserve the patient's autonomy in the therapeutic situation, the analyst must avoid all unnecessary coercion. Since the only thing the analyst really needs (or ought to need) is money, the only legitimate demand on the patient is money. Indeed, what other demands can the analyst, as an autonomous therapist, have? Surely he cannot require the patient to lie on the couch or free-associate, to refrain from sexual misbehavior or law-breaking, or any of the myriad things that therapists demand from their patients.

Like everyone else, the analyst is a real person; he has real needs. But in analysis he can expect the patient to satisfy *only one* of his needs, namely, his need for money. Practicing analysis is a profession; it is the way the analyst makes a living. This is why it is "realistic," psychologically and socially, for the patient to pay the analyst.

If the analyst expects the patient to satisfy other needs, he vitiates the analysis. For example, the therapist may have a need to be a good parent, to be loved and admired, to be forgiving, to succor the weak, to make secret alliances with patients against the outside world, to play doctor, to remake personalities, and so on. But why expect the analysand to satisfy them? In my opinion, the patient should no more satisfy any of these (or other) needs than he ought to satisfy, for example, the analyst's craving for sexual pleasure. The therapist must fulfill his aspirations and needs through objects other than the patient. I repeat, the analysand owes *only* money to the analyst. Needless to say, the patient's self-transformation will cost him more than just money; but the extra cost is not payable to the analyst.

The stipulation that the analysand be deprived of certain opportunities to satisfy the needs of the analyst may also be the source of difficulties; it is necessary to understand these and guard against them. For example, the analyst may come to believe that he "gives" too much to the patient and "receives" nothing from him in return; this will make the therapist feel bountiful and magnanimous and, reactively, perhaps demanding as well. The situation is comparable to certain relations between child and parent or between husband and wife where each feels either exploited by his partner or guilty toward him. How can we avoid this?

The best safeguard is the economic basis of the analytic relationship. The analyst usually needs the money that the patient pays him. For the therapist, the fee is tangible evidence that he "receives" something from the patient; he will therefore be less likely to feel exploited (especially if he considers the fee high enough). However, for the money transaction to have the significance I am here attributing to it, the analyst must feel comfortable about it. If he denies or minimizes what money means to him, he will deprive the patient of paying him with money *only* and will burden the patient with expectations of other kinds of "payment." If, on the other hand, the analyst overvalues money, he will make other mistakes. Fearful of losing the patient, he will set his fee too low and resent it. Greedy to make as much as possible, he will set his fee too high, and his patient will resent it. Or the analyst will abandon analysis altogether and sell the patient whatever he seems to want to buy.

If the analytic contract is properly negotiated, the fee should satisfy both parties. The analyst ought to feel that he is well paid for his services, and the analysand, that he owes the analyst only money and only as much as he can afford. Again, this has certain practical implications. The contract for the fee—or, more generally, for the amount the patient owes the analyst—is often broken in two ways. First, the analysand may refuse to pay or be delinquent in paying; if the analyst does not stop the treatment but reduces the fee or lets the patient accumulate a debt, he will have ended the analytic relationship and created instead a psychotherapeutic situation that is neither analytic nor autonomous. Second, in response to the analyst's expectations or from his own motives, the analysand may wish to do more for the analyst than pay his fee (e.g., finance his research, give him valuable gifts, and so forth); if the analyst lets the patient over-fulfill his contract, he will have succeeded in destroying the analytic relationship.*

The conditions that I have outlined are those of successful analysis; they create an atmosphere in which the patient realizes that the therapy is his, not someone else's. On the other hand, if the therapist lays down various rules—such as requiring the patient to lie on the couch, to free-associate, to report his dreams—he inevitably creates a situation in which the patient can cooperate or refuse to cooperate, can be a good patient or bad patient, and so forth.

All these possibilities and the complications that result from them are avoided if the analyst renounces the traditional role of doctor or therapist who tries to do a job *on* the patient or *on* his sickness. Instead, by adopting the role of expert who sells his services and becomes contractually obligated to his client, the therapist retains just enough power to discharge his duty, that is, to play the role of analyst. The therapist needs no power beyond this, for it is not necessary for him to judge whether the client is a good or bad patient or to participate as an authority in the client's extra-analytic life; indeed, the possession of such power interferes with the performance of the analytic task.

* See Chapter 13.

The Integrity of the Analytic Relationship

The rules of the analytic game serve a single, basic aim: to preserve the integrity of the analytic relationship. It is impossible to play contract bridge if one of the players is allowed to cheat because he complains of a headache. In proportion as a contract can be broken, it is not a contract. This and this alone is why the analyst must eschew the roles of doctor and psychiatrist. These are status roles, not contract roles; they give their bearers the right and indeed the responsibility to take matters into their own hands and, if necessary, "save the patient from himself." But, if the analyst wants to save a patient from himself, he cannot analyze that patient. Otherwise it is a mockery to speak of the patient as an autonomous agent. A great many people *are* able and willing to conduct themselves as self-responsible analytic patients, but the therapist can never discover who they are unless he himself acts autonomously, that is, contractually.

The therapist who is comfortable in the role I have indicated will find many patients who not only accept this arrangement but like it. This need not surprise us. Patients who consult analysts often want analysis, not something else. Accordingly, they are pleased to find an analyst who sells analysis, not something else. Many patients do not want the psychotherapist to do things other than psychotherapy. However, they become confused when the therapist seems willing, indeed eager, to perform other activities as well. Thus, complications in psychotherapy arise not so much from the patient's demands for nonpsychological interventions as from the therapist's eagerness to play doctor.

To be sure, some patients may not wish to buy a purely psychotherapeutic or analytic product. The therapist's obligation is to make clear what he sells. If the patient wishes some other type of therapeutic commodity, he will soon stop seeing the analyst and perhaps seek another therapist. If, however, the arrangement seems satisfactory to him, it will be so without the therapist having made any false representations.

The autonomous therapist offers to sell *only* his skills as an analyst. If the patient is sick, he must consult a physician; if he wishes to obtain drugs, he must do so from someone other than the analyst; and so forth. Some analysts do indeed conduct themselves in this way. Many others, however, do not; they prescribe drugs and even use convulsive therapy, while "analyzing" the patient. They justify this dilution of the analytic role by claiming that the patient "needs" such adjuvant therapies and by asserting that they are, after all, physicians and should therefore offer the patient all their medical skills. This is nonsense.

To be sure, the therapist has every right to practice in this way. If his patients benefit, the therapist's reward will be a lucrative practice. Nevertheless, the foregoing argument is nonsensical or worse because it undermines the analytic contract and thus destroys psychoanalysis as autonomous psychotherapy. We may grant the claim that the patient in analysis may need drugs and many other things as well. My point is this: if the therapist is to do his job as analyst correctly and well, he cannot provide other services. Nor does he need to; the patient is free to secure them from others.

The additional argument that the analyst is a physician and hence owes the patient the full range of his knowledge and skills is absurd. The therapist owes the patient no more and certainly no less than what he contracts for; if he promises the patient only psychotherapy, he owes him only psychotherapy. Furthermore, the fact that the therapist is a physician is largely a historical accident; his medical training and credentials help him little, if at all, with his task as psychotherapist.

It is also possible that the therapist possesses skills additional and quite unrelated to those of analyst and physician. For example, the therapist may be an expert bridge-player, accomplished musician, or experienced investor in the stock market. Suppose the analysand wishes to take advantage of one of these skills? Will the analyst teach the patient how to play bridge, play the piano, or make money in the stock market? If he lends the patient his medical skills, why not lend him his other skills? I mention this line of reasoning, not only to clarify this issue, but also to suggest an explanation that may help some patients to understand why the analyst refuses to help in any way except by analyzing. The limitation of the analyst's role may disappoint the patient. But it is only the disappointment not dispelled by such realistic explanations that can be subjected to fruitful analytic scrutiny.

9

The Terminal Period

THE TRADITIONAL ANALYTIC VIEW OF TERMINATION

LET us review the principles for ending autonomous psychotherapy against the backdrop of established psychoanalytic theory. However much psychoanalytic therapy may differ from other forms of psychiatric treatment, the analyst's concept of his role as therapist resembles the traditional medical view of the doctor's role. Thus, the analyst has accepted the basic premises of the sickness-healing model: the patient is ill; the therapist makes a diagnosis, carries out the treatment, decides when the patient is well, and discharges him from therapy.

With minor variations, this theme has been applied by psychoanalytic theoreticians to the analytic situation: the analysand presents himself to the analyst with a mental disturbance; the analyst diagnoses the disturbance, and, if it is an appropriate neurosis (that is, if the patient is analyzable), he embarks on an analysis. The patient develops a transference neurosis, which is subjected to systematic analysis; when the transference neurosis is adequately analyzed, the therapeutic relationship is terminated by the analyst.

There is much that is valuable in this schematic view of the analytic process, but the spirit that it inspires is false. It suggests that analysis is a process of recovery from illness, rather than an enterprise in education and self-transformation, and that, just as the medical patient's recovery from illness is judged by the physician, so the analytic patient's recovery from neurosis is judged by the therapist. Hence, the analyst should play a major role in deciding when therapy should be terminated. Analysts usually do this, yet their doing so is utterly opposed to the aim and spirit of analysis as autonomous therapy.

Because analytic theorists base their reasoning on the medical model, they seek quasimedical, psychopathological criteria for their decision to terminate treatment. This is a dilemma that analysts have never been able to resolve adequately. I hold that the analyst has no right to terminate the analysis. This is not his job; it is the patient's. It is hardly surprising, then, that the voluminous literature on the so-called problem of termination is a mass of confusion.

The effort to establish psychodynamic criteria for termination is comparable to the effort to establish criteria for analyzability. The therapist who wishes to ascertain whether a patient is analyzable is, in effect, trying to predict the patient's future behavior. But there is no good reason why he should do this. Instead of trying to find out whether the patient is analyzable, the therapist need only determine whether he wants to buy his services. If the patient is not analyzable, both therapist and patient will discover this as they become better acquainted. To repeat, there is no valid reason for the analyst to try to predict the patient's behavior. Instead, he ought to inform the patient of his—the analyst's—future behavior, governed by the rules of analysis.

If the therapist accepts responsibility for terminating therapy (as he does for starting it, when he tries to assess the patient's analyzability), he must have some rational basis for deciding when to end it. Moreover, the analyst is not free to search for a suitable basis for this decision; his traditional conceptual model compels him to base this judgment on the analysand's psychic condition. From this point of view, therefore, the patient's decision to stop is not an adequate reason for doing so. From my point of view, it is.

As we know, it is difficult to assess another person's "mental state." Nevertheless, the analyst places himself in the position of assuming that some mental states are indications for stopping analysis, but that others are not, and he accepts the responsibility for making these "diagnostic" evaluations and for acting on them.

The results have been disastrous. Theoretically, a plethora of criteria for termination have been suggested. Practically, the method of ending the analysis has been shrouded in mystery. The suspicion lingers that the analyst's criteria for termination and the actual ending of analysis are only remotely connected. To be sure, it is often stated that the analytic criteria for termination describe ideal conditions which the patient is expected to approximate but can rarely attain. But this is evasion. The facts remain that standards for ending the analysis have been created and that analysts match the behavior of their patients against them. But we ought to question the legitimacy and value of the analyst's diagnostic evaluation of the analysand.

What are the criteria for termination? The following have been suggested by leading analysts: (1) attainment by the patient of the genital stage of psychosexual development; (2) development of the patient to emotional maturity; (3) adequate analysis and resolution of the transference neurosis; (4) adequate analysis of the patient's "depressive and schizoid positions"; (5) "structural change" in the patient's personality. (Neo-Freudian analysts have added other criteria.)

Some of these concepts are more meaningful and useful than others. In particular, the analysis of the transference neurosis is a valuable concept; but what constitutes an "adequate" analysis of it is another matter. Yet, however meaningful or meaningless these terms may be—and analysts differ on this—their value for the kind of decision-making we are considering is limited.

THE ROLES OF THE PAST AND OF THE FUTURE IN THERAPEUTIC DECISION-MAKING

We are concerned now with the following questions: How does the physician ascertain the nature of the patient's illness and the treatment to apply? How does the psychoanalyst assume a similar responsibility for deciding when to begin and when to terminate an analysis?

The physician uses three methods for making a diagnosis: he takes the history of the patient's illness, examines the patient's body, and tests his bodily functions with various special procedures. The first of these methods—which for centuries was the physician's principal technique for ascertaining the nature of the patient's ailment—relies entirely on past events; the two others assess current events.

It is often assumed that decision about medical therapy flows logically from medical diagnosis. Sometimes it seems to. However, this assumption obscures the important role of anticipated future events in decisions about treatment. The conscientious physician and the intelligent patient will want to know, not only what ails the patient, but also what will help or harm him. Thus, in deciding about therapy, they also consider the future.

In general, the physician looks mainly to the past if his work is diagnostic, to the future if it is therapeutic. Thus, when a person is ill and consults a physician, he is often concerned about the nature of his illness: What is it? Is it contagious? Hereditary? Serious? On the other hand, when a skier with a broken ankle consults an orthopedic surgeon, he is concerned about the nature and prospects of the therapy: How long will my ankle be in a cast? When can I ski again? Since the diagnosis is obvious in this type of case, decision-making centers on the prospects of the therapy.

As a rule, the prospective analytic patient is like this kind of medical patient; the "diagnosis" is obvious and hence not an issue. In a fundamental sense, the person seeking analytic help makes his own diagnosis: he suffers from hypochondriacal anxieties, is unhappily married and cannot extricate himself from the situation, is homosexual, and so forth. The patient knows what ails him; indeed, he defines himself as "sick," in the sense of needing psychotherapeutic help. Accordingly, the patient is not primarily concerned about the nature of his difficulty, but rather about the possibilities of overcoming it: Would psychoanalysis help? How long would it take? How much would it cost?

Thus, the prospective analysand focuses on the future. However, the analyst practicing in a traditional fashion, feeling obliged to ascertain whether the patient is analyzable, will focus on the past. The patient wants to know what *will* happen to him (in analysis), whereas the analyst wants to know what *has* happened to him (in his childhood). Hence, the interests of analyst and analysand are likely to conflict soon after they meet. As I have indicated, moreover, the patient's history, no matter how accurately elicited, provides insufficient evidence for this sort of decision-making.

In contrast to the traditional analyst, the autonomous psychotherapist deals with the problem of analyzability by letting the patient assume responsibility for deciding whether he wishes to be analyzed; he then bases his own judgments—necessary for determining whether to accept the patient as an analysand—not on the patient's past history, but rather on his current behavior in the trial phase of therapy.

Solution of the problem of how to terminate analysis may be sought in the same way. I submit that the therapist need not, indeed should not, assume responsibility for terminating therapy. Although the decision to end the analysis must rest with the patient, this does not mean that the analyst may not express his views on this subject. What are the criteria for his opinions?

Again we should consider a change in our usual time perspective on this matter. At the beginning of treatment, the therapist should not focus on the past; instead, he should keep the past and the future at the periphery of his attention and place the present in the center. When contemplating termination, the therapist should not focus on the past and the present, but on the future. The important questions at this time are not: "What has been accomplished?" or "Has this or that problem been sufficiently analyzed?", but rather: "What else or what more does the patient want to gain from treatment?" or "Does the analyst believe that he can continue to render service to the patient?"

My views on the practical aspects of terminating autonomous psychotherapy are presented in Chapter 15. Some further remarks on the principles underlying the ending of the treatment are in order here.

PRINCIPLES FOR TERMINATING ANALYSIS AUTONOMOUSLY

The fundamental aim of analysis is to enlarge the patient's capacity for making decisions. Accordingly, the analyst must scrupulously avoid interfering with or usurping the patient's responsibility for choosing between alternative courses of action. Decisions about the treatment itself—that is, whether to begin analysis, continue, or terminate it—are among the important decisions for the analysand to make. Should the therapist make them for him, the very idea of autonomous therapy would be a mockery. Such a therapeutic situation would be comparable to a relationship between father and son where the father asserts that his son is free to spend his savings as he pleases, but in fact interferes whenever he disapproves.

Let us recall one of the most significant aspects of the therapeutic contract which is undertaken by analysand and analyst at end of the trial period: the therapist renounces the physician's traditional option of discharging the patient from therapy (except for nonpayment of the fee). Hence, the analyst has no pressing need to determine when the patient is "cured" and ready to be discharged from therapy. Indeed, his contract with the analysand explicitly forbids this.

Some may object that this is unmedical and "untherapeutic." It is, and for good reason. The analyst negotiates a contract with the patient and must uphold its terms. He must neither default on his promises nor fulfill obligations he has not incurred. The analyst does not promise to cure the patient, to formulate standards of adequate mental health for him, or to decide when therapy should be terminated. Accordingly the analyst need not and, indeed, must not grapple with the question of ending analysis. That is the patient's problem. How could it be anyone else's? What legitimate interest can the analyst have in continuing or terminating the treatment?

The Medical Game and Its Rules for Termination

Again we must first consider the medical situation. For the doctor, it would be questionable practice to continue treating a patient and accepting his money for doing so well past the time when he no longer needs medical assistance. In part, then, it is a problem of medical ethics. But that is not all.

The busy physician likes to be usefully employed. This wish gives him a personal incentive, independent of the financial one, to devote his time and energy to sick patients—perhaps to them only. Here is where the medical game becomes more complicated. The "busy" doctor may become like the mother of a large family who must withdraw care from the older children and devote herself to the younger ones. However, if the physician is free to decide that patient A, who has recovered or nearly recovered, needs him less than patient B, who is ill, what is to prevent him from declaring that patient C is incurable and hence less deserving of his attention than patient D, who is only slightly ill but likely to recover? And what happens when a new patient appears who offers to pay more than any of the physician's current patients? Will the doctor be tempted to feel that here, at last, is an especially interesting and meritorious case? Clearly, there are all sorts of possibilities for arbitrary (and venal) actions by physicians who play according to these rules of the medical game.

The Analytic Game and Its Rules for Termination

Let us recall three basic rules of the analytic game. First, the analyst, unlike the physician, is not engaged in the business of healing sickness; second, his relationship with the patient is regulated by contract, not by the patient's real or alleged needs; third, the analyst does not discharge the patient when cured. Were he to retain this option, it would tend to vitiate his entire "therapeutic" effort. Curiously, the last-mentioned phenomenon has escaped the attention of psychiatrists and psychoanalysts.

Why must the analyst renounce the option of severing the therapeutic relationship? Before we can answer this question, we must briefly reconstruct the essential features of the analytic situation. If patient and analyst proceed to the contractual phase, we may assume that each considers the other a worthwhile person. The patient will come to trust the analyst and will confide his most embarrassing secrets to him. It is necessary and useful for the patient to do so, for this is the road to self-discovery and increased self-responsibility. Accordingly, the analyst must foster those conditions that facilitate the patient's frank self-disclosure and guard against those that tend to inhibit it. Nothing inhibits a person's frankness more effectively than the fear that his confidences will be used against him. Thus, the analyst guarantees the patient that all his communications—not just his secrets— will be kept absolutely private. But there are other hazards to self-disclosure.

Because of the nature of the analytic relationship, therapy becomes important to the patient in proportion to his commitment to it. This becomes related to his fear of losing the analytic relationship. How can the patient lose this important "object"?

First, the analyst may become ill, die, or move to another city. There is not much that either analyst or patient can do about such things. (However, if a therapist expects to leave a city or for some other reason be available to a patient for a limited time only, he should not accept patients for long-term psychotherapy.)

Second, the analyst may decide to alter, interrupt, or terminate therapy. Why should he do any of these things? Like the medical doctor, the analyst, too, may prefer to treat only "sick people," possibly only "very sick people." If this is so, his analysand will be threatened by any progress in the analysis, for he will be "rewarded" for it by being abandoned by the analyst in favor of a psychologically more disabled patient. Or the analyst may wish to make more money, and a patient able to pay a higher fee may request therapy. If the analyst's schedule is full, how could he make room for him? By concluding that one of his analysands has recovered sufficiently to terminate. Or the analyst may have grown tired of a patient. Might he not be tempted to conclude that the analysand is incurable or at least not further analyzable by him and so rid himself of a difficult patient?

There are many other possibilities. An important one is that the analyst, because of the patient's self-disclosures, may feel ill disposed toward him, at least during certain periods. Patients almost invariably fear that their self-betrayals will alienate their analysts and result in the termination of their treatment.

These hazards are inherent in the psychotherapeutic relationship. For the autonomous therapist, there is only one remedy for them: to place the therapy squarely in the hands of the patient to do with as he sees fit (within the limits of the contract). This means that the analyst (and, to a lesser extent, the patient) must relinquish the option to tamper with the treatment; he cannot reduce the hours, increase the fee, interrupt or stop the treatment, and so forth.

Each of these potential moves in the psychotherapy game can serve as a powerful weapon in the hands of the therapist. Thus, if the therapist wants to ensure favorable conditions for the patient to learn about himself and his relationship to others and to develop his autonomy, he must relinquish what are, in effect, weapons against the patient. Only when the therapist renounces the traditional privileges of the physician is the patient genuinely free to use the treatment for his own self-development. Indeed, when analysis is so structured, there is nothing else that the analysand can use it for!

On Terminating Games: Implications of the Bridge Model

I have used the model of contract bridge to shed light on the nature of the therapeutic collaboration between analyst and analysand. The trial period is like bidding; the players negotiate a contract. The contractual phase is like playing one's cards; the high bidder does the work necessary for fulfilling the contract. Does this model increase our understanding of the problem of terminating analytic treatment? I think that it does.

The game of contract bridge is composed of units: a single contract, a game, and a rubber. Thus, the rubber is the whole, and contracts and games are parts. The discussion, clarification, and interpretation of particular topics, problems, or transference phenomena are like the play of hands and the completion of games and rubbers. With each, the game advances. But there is nothing in the rules of either bridge or psychoanalysis that can tell us when the partnership of two bridge-players or of analyst and analysand should end. These are *decisions* made by the participants. To be sure, some situations provide more reasonable stopping places than others. But this "reasonableness" of the breaking-off point is a human decision, and players in a game or analyst and patient may agree or disagree.

In the case of bridge, the players may have decided at the start to complete one of several rubbers before stopping. However, when the play is informal, the game may come to a halt at any time. In autonomous psychotherapy, the participants make a prior agreement about the duration of the treatment; contingent on the patient's proper conduct, the therapist must stay in the game indefinitely! In this, the analyst's obligation is comparable to that of the bank in Monte Carlo (or in other honestly run gaming establishments): the customer *may* start or stop playing as he chooses; the bank *must* play. Except for holidays and certain hours of the day when it closes, the casino must stay open for business. It cannot stop accepting bets when it is losing heavily, although the customer may leave after winning a large sum. But, even with these concessions, over the long run the bank is in a more favorable position to win than are the customers. These considerations also help explain why roulette is a game only for the person who bets, but business for the croupier and the owner of the establishment.

The same distinction applies to analysand and analyst. To the former, analysis is a part-time activity, not quite real, carefully separated from the rest of his life. To the latter, it is an occupation, wholly real, a large and integral part of his life. Thus the analysand can leave the patient role and continue to live his real, extra-analytic life; the analyst cannot give up the therapist role without changing occupation. The reality or businesslike character for the analyst of the analytic game has far-reaching implications for his life. These are, however, not germane to the present discussion.

We should realize clearly that, in discussing termination, we are asking a question, not about the game, but about the length of time the players should continue to play. The structure of games does not generally provide an answer to this. How many rubbers two bridge-players play depends, not on the game, but on them. Some bridge teams continue in active partnership for years and decades; others last only an evening or the fraction of an hour. Who is to say, except the players themselves, how long they ought to play together? There are always new hands to be dealt, a new contract to be bid and fulfilled. In principle, a bridge partnership is of indefinite duration. In practice, the duration of the game (in this extended sense) depends on the partners' decision to continue or discontinue the relationship; the game ends when the relationship ends.

I think that we ought to have a similar view of the analytic relationship. In bridge, there is always another hand to play. In analysis, there is always more that could be said about the patient's childhood, the analytic situation, and, last but not least, about the patient's current situation; like new deals in a card game, the latter is an endless source of new "reality problems." Who is to say when these topics and problems are exhausted and hence that the game is over? There is nothing and there can be nothing in the rules of the analytic game to command the players to stop playing. When to bring the enterprise to a halt must be decided by the players, alone or together. For reasons mentioned earlier, it is necessary that the analyst promise not to discontinue the game as long as the patient wishes to play. This does not mean that the analyst cannot raise the question of stopping and suggest reasons for and against doing so. Nor does it mean that, although the final decision is in the hands of the patient, analyst and analysand cannot cooperate in reaching the decision. Ideally, analysis ought to be terminated as other co-operative games or ventures are, by the mutual consent of the partners.

Autonomy, Liberty, and Psychotherapy

These principles for terminating autonomous psychotherapy are logically consistent, psychologically sound, and faithful to the ethics of autonomy. No patient can be considered autonomous if what he reveals about himself threatens the therapeutic relationship. A person is free only when he knows the circumstances under which he will be penalized; he can maintain his liberty by not engaging in acts that are prohibited. The analytic contract must promise nothing less. Indeed, why should it? Why should the analyst wish to retain the privilege of ending the analysis, especially on the ground that he is acting in the patient's best interests?

When the analyst is at the threshold of committing himself to a contractual relationship with the patient, he must ask himself this question: "What kind of relationship do I want to have with the patient?" As analyst, the therapist must make an indefinite time commitment to the patient. If he does not care to do this with a particular patient, it would be wiser not to accept him for analysis; and, if he does not want to do it at all, he should not become an analyst. In part, the problem centers once more on the therapist's personality and interests. If he is interested in analysis and likes doing this sort of work, he will not wish to be coercive. Indeed, he will realize that, for the analyst, power over the patient—whether to order him about or to terminate his treatment—is a hindrance, not a help.

In human affairs, power and understanding are antithetical to each other. The psychotherapist must choose between controlling his patient and sharing information with him. If he chooses control, he will have little need for understanding (although he may wish to clothe his coercive tactics in pseudo-scientific rationalizations). As history shows, to control people, we must enslave them, and, to maintain control, we must curtail their access to information.

Despite the inverse relation between man's wish to control his fellow man and his wish to understand him, psychotherapists seem to have wanted the best of two incompatible worlds. They have tried to combine understanding the patient with controlling him (allegedly in his own best interests). Analysts have thus sought to control man on the basis of an allegedly scientific understanding of his behavior. But this is absurd, because, as suggested, the more we want to control another person's conduct, the less we need to understand it.

Finally, the inverse relation between power and understanding accounts for the fact that, the more intimately we understand a person, the more difficult it is to control him; our very understanding inhibits us from influencing him forcefully. Indeed, we can understand another person only in proportion to our willingness to restrain ourselves from dominating him or submitting to him. Conversely, if we wish to dominate others (whether individuals or groups), it is easier to do so if we can declare them alien or subhuman, in brief, beyond the pale of our understanding. This is the typical posture of those who wish to control and oppress the members of alien races, mental patients, or political enemies.

In sum, if the therapist truly desires to liberate the patient, to help him become *personally free*, he must arrange a therapeutic situation where such freedom can develop and flourish. In this, his role is comparable to that of the legislator. The founding fathers desired to create a society of free men. Wanting to make it possible for people to be *politically free*, they tried to provide a political situation where such freedom could develop and flourish. The Constitution of the United States is a contract between the American people and their governors to ensure political freedom. To this end, the government agrees to renounce such traditional rights of governors as torturing subjects, trying them in secret and by their adversaries, searching their premises and persons at will, requiring them to incriminate themselves or suffer the consequences, and other methods for maintaining social order.

I conceive the analytic contract in similar terms. It guarantees the patient certain rights absent in the traditional physician–patient relationship. As a result, the patient acquires an opportunity to become personally free and incurs an obligation to conduct himself responsibly.

III

THE METHOD OF

AUTONOMOUS

PSYCHOTHERAPY

10

The Initial Contact between

Patient and Therapist

THE PRINCIPLE OF AUTONOMY AND THE PSYCHOANALYTIC METHOD

GAIUS, the famous Roman jurist, said that the principal part of everything is the beginning. This is especially true of the psychoanalytic relationship.

The early stages of the therapeutic encounter are crucial; slight errors on the part of the therapist may destroy the developing analytic relationship or prevent it from becoming truly analytic and autonomous. Thus, the manner in which patient and psychotherapist first meet and the nature of their initial communications with each other are exceptionally important.

It is the therapist's, not the patient's, initial conduct that constitutes the significant opening move in the therapeutic game. Once a certain kind of therapeutic climate is established, it may be difficult or impossible to alter. Indeed, the question immediately arises: Why should one kind of game be first established, only to be altered subsequently? Accordingly, if the therapist intends to practice autonomous psychotherapy, the time to begin is when he first makes contact with the patient.

The psychoanalyst's conduct must flow directly from his commitment to the ethic of autonomy. Although never clearly articulated in theory, this idea is not entirely new in analytic practice. For example, it is part of the folklore of psychoanalytic technique that the analyst insist that the patient himself make the initial appointment. If someone else contacts the analyst, he should be asked to request the patient to call. This is sound advice, although often justified on false or misleading grounds, for example, as a good method for weeding out poorly motivated patients. Though the practice may help accomplish this, it is not the main reason for it. In my opinion the only adequate justification for this rule (and for most others in analysis) is that it maintains or enhances the autonomy of the participants in the relationship.

There is no place in analysis for the therapist who likes to play the standard role of the busy, important professional man who delegates as much work as possible to secretaries and other assistants. Thus, the analyst cannot entrust to others the setting and collection of the fee; he must discuss and establish it with the patient and also accept payment directly from him. I believe that this practice is often followed. But, once again, the reason for it is not only because the financial transaction between analyst and analysand is an integral part of the analysis, but rather because a third party in this transaction would detract needlessly from the autonomous positions of the participants.

Similar considerations hold for making appointments. The autonomous therapist must do this himself. This need not be a rigid rule; rather, it is a methodological principle, firmly based on theory. The scheduling of appointments is the sole concern of the therapist and the patient. Third parties must be barred from it to protect the autonomy of the participants and the privacy of the situation. It is absurd, therefore, for the therapist to insist that his potential patient make his own initial appointment and then delegate some part of the arrangement to his secretary. It is even more absurd for the analyst to delegate to his secretary the task of negotiating appointments with a patient who is in treatment.

In sum, the analyst's obligation to act autonomously is far-reaching, whereas the analysand's is limited.

How Does a Person Become a Psychotherapy Patient?

The psychotherapist's services are usually solicited in one of the following ways. First, the prospective client may call for an appointment. Second, a relative or friend of the patient may call. Third, the patient may be referred by a professional colleague (physician, psychologist, college professor, etc.), he or his secretary calling for the appointment. Fourth, such persons in social authority as attorneys, judges, probation officers, school officials, or social workers may contact the therapist, ostensibly in behalf of the patient and for the purpose of making an appointment for him.

Regardless of who contacts the therapist (or his office), the analyst should speak to the caller himself or, if busy, should return the call at his earliest convenience. To anyone but the patient, the analyst will explain that he will be glad to talk to the patient about scheduling an appointment. If the caller wants to explain why this is impossible, the therapist must listen politely but must stand firm; he may, if he wishes, offer a counterargument. For example, the caller may assert that the patient is "too nervous" or "too upset" and has therefore requested his wife (father, etc.) to call for him; the therapist may point out that the patient will have to talk to him during an appointment and question the purpose of making one if the patient cannot even converse on the telephone. In this way, the therapist will also convey to those who call something about his work.

This kind of initial clarification can prevent a host of misunderstandings which are likely to arise if the therapist lets the patient or whoever calls for him keep his image of the therapist and of the work he does. If the therapist establishes some initial rules at the outset, he will eliminate as patients those who wish to play games in which the therapist does not want to participate.

These principles apply also to referrals from physicians. Fearful of losing such referrals and hence suffering economically, psychotherapists often make a mistake in this sort of situation. For example, the referring physician may have his secretary call to make an appointment for a patient. But the psychoanalyst cannot follow this medical routine and still practice autonomous therapy with the patient so referred. Instead, he must explain the reasons for his rules about scheduling appointments and confidentiality to his medical colleagues. Then, if the referring physician wishes to recommend to his patient that he consult a psychoanalyst—rather than, say, a psychiatrist who uses mainly drugs and shock treatment or who practices group therapy and family counseling—he will not object to letting the patient call for his own appointment.

If, on the other hand, the referring physician is contemptuous of these rules, he is likely to try to cope with those patients who could benefit from analysis and use referral to the psychiatrist mainly as a means of punishing the patient. Clearly, under these circumstances, the autonomous psychotherapist cannot enter into a cooperative arrangement with a medical colleague.

Finally, a representative of a social agency or institution may call to make an appointment for someone defined as a patient. Here, too, the therapist may elect to explain his rules to the caller. Or, if it is clear that the caller is not seeking a psychiatrist who will do something *for* the patient but rather one who will do something *to* him, it may be better for the analyst to explain that this is not the sort of psychiatry he practices and abort the relationship before it begins.

CLARIFICATIONS BEFORE THE INITIAL APPOINTMENT

The first contact between client and therapist is usually a telephone conversation. The patient may give his name and ask for an appointment. Should the therapist respond with an offer of a time for an appointment so that he and the patient can schedule their first meeting? Though this may seem to be common sense, it may be a mistake to follow it. Even before a therapeutic relationship is established, we must recognize and utilize one of the basic principles of autonomous psychotherapy: the therapist must never mislead the patient. One of the most effective ways for the therapist to discharge this obligation is to clarify *his own* position, so far as it may affect the patient. In practice, this means several things.

For example, the therapist's schedule may be full. He may therefore be unable to accept a new patient for analysis, but may still see patients for evaluation, clarification of problems, referral to colleagues, or for placement on his waiting list. A person is entitled to this information when he calls. If it is withheld and the patient given an appointment, he may gain the impression that he has taken the first step toward the beginning of an analysis when in fact he has not.

If the analyst cannot accept a new patient for intensive therapy, he should find out what the patient wants when he is asking for an appointment. If the answer is analysis (or words to that effect), the therapist should explain that his schedule for analytic work is full. This exchange on the telephone will save both patient and analyst a great deal of trouble. It will also distinguish those who are looking for help from *analysis* (or some other form of psychotherapy) from those who are looking for help from a particular *analyst*.

Why all this fuss? The patient has asked for an appointment, not for an analysis; why not simply give him an appointment? The reasons (and I have already suggested some) are obvious. However, since the practice of acquainting the patient with the therapist's actual situation and methods is not generally accepted, these questions deserve explicit answers.

The patient may not be clear about the work methods of the analyst. Even if he is, he may be reticent about asking the analyst questions before meeting him. In any case, if the patient receives an appointment, visits the therapist, and is *then* told that the therapist has no time to accept new patients, his first experience with psychotherapy will be noxious, not therapeutic. Such a patient will believe, rightly, that he should have been told this on the telephone, not in the consulting room; it would have saved him time, anguish, and money.

Worse yet, the patient may conclude that the therapist is lying about not having time. Therapists often proffer this reason for not accepting a patient for therapy, when actually it is not the reason. The patient may believe that he is not accepted for treatment because he is unanalyzable, psychotic, or something of the sort, and he cannot be blamed for drawing such inferences, however false they may be. Lack of therapeutic time can be an acceptable reason for "rejecting" a patient only if he is informed about it before the therapist sets eyes on him. Once the two have met, the patient cannot be expected to believe that the therapist's decision is not based, at least partly, on the therapist's impressions of the patient.

Sometimes a patient sees several therapists, telling each something about himself, only to be informed that the therapist has no time to accept him as a patient. After one or more such experiences, the patient is likely to ask the analyst, while still on the telephone, whether he has time for therapy. But by then much harm may have been done; the patient has already learned to expect the analyst to withhold facts that vitally concern him, as his parents might have when he was a child. In sum, I submit that, if the therapist cannot accept new patients for therapy, he has every reason to tell this to prospective patients and no valid reason not to.

If the analyst has free time and the patient merely asks for an appointment, the situation may not require further discussion. However, if the analyst has reason to think that the patient wants to be analyzed or the patient informs him that he does, further clarification of the situation may again avert later difficulties and misunderstandings. I usually tell the prospective patient that I do have time for a new patient (if I do and if this question is at issue), but that I cannot decide to undertake an analysis without a good deal of contact with him. If the patient is still interested, I suggest making an appointment to discuss the matter in person.

There are many questions patients may ask while still on the telephone, before making their first appointment. What is the analyst's fee? What is his religion? How long will the analysis last? Does the analyst practice hypnosis? Will the analysis help? Does the analyst recommend it? And so on. How should the therapist deal with such questions? On what basis or principle should he decide whether to answer questions and, if to answer, which ones?

Many analysts avoid answering all such questions. This is, I believe, a mistake. Others, using intuition as their standard of judgment, answer some questions but not others. This is a little better, but not good enough. Is there a criterion for deciding which of the patient's questions deserve an honest and factual answer? Our criterion should be the relevance of the question to the therapeutic situation. Pertinent questions should be answered, but not others.

If the patient asks about the fee, there can be no justification for evasion or refusal to answer. If he asks about the analyst's religion, national origin, or membership in one or another professional organization, again I think that the therapist ought to give simple, factual answers; these questions seek information that may assist the prospective client to decide whether to undertake treatment with him. If the aim of psychoanalysis is to help the patient maximize his choices in the conduct of his life, how can we, by withholding information from him, interfere with his making self-responsible decisions? Or, to put it differently, how can we expect the patient to conduct himself autonomously, when, at the very beginning of our relationship with him, we make it impossible for him to behave that way toward us?

Of course, there is another type of question—such as "Will the analysis help?"—that does not meet the criterion. Questions like this should not be answered. However, even in these cases, the analyst should not be evasive, but should say frankly: "I don't know" or "I can't answer that question."

Finally, there is a third type of question, such as "Are you married?" or "Do you have children?" These pertain to what the analyst, though not necessarily the patient, may consider personal matters unrelated to the therapeutic situation. I believe that the response should be something like: "I prefer not to answer that." Undoubtedly, there are differences among therapists over certain questions, some believing that the inquiries pertain to matters affecting the patient's "realistic" position in the therapeutic situation; others, that they represent merely "curiosity" about the analyst. In the long run, such differences do not matter. What does is that the analyst have some clear ideas on these issues and, further, that he indicate to the patient, by candidly answering some questions but not others, that the patient is entitled (a) to ask anything and (b) to receive frank and factual answers to questions that affect him in his role as analysand, but not to those that seek to satisfy his curiosity about the analyst.

The methodological principles that I have outlined apply, not only to the first telephone conversation between patient and therapist, but also to the therapeutic situation that may subsequently develop.

THE INITIAL INTERVIEWS

The purpose of the first, or preliminary, interviews is to provide the client and the therapist with an opportunity to get acquainted. In other words, the autonomous therapist must discover what the client wishes to buy and inform the client what he is offering to sell. Let us review some of the specific actions in this initial phase of therapy.

After entering the therapist's office, the client is offered a seat, either in a chair or on a couch equipped with a backrest. The therapist sits facing the patient, not too far from him. More than six or eight feet between the participants creates an atmosphere of "distance." So does placing a desk or other furniture between therapist and client.

The therapist's demeanor, like the decoration of the office, should be something between stern aloofness and excessive friendliness. The occasion calls for a combination of kindness and professional objectivity. After putting the patient at ease, the therapist should indicate that all his attention is directed to the patient and his problems.

I find it useful to begin with a question like, "What brings you here?" or "What can I do for you?" I pause and let the patient speak. Without questions or prompting, many patients present a detailed and meaningful account of the circumstances from which they seek release. Others answer my initial question briefly, naming only some symptom or acute problem and then waiting for me to participate more actively.

What about the patient who finds it difficult to begin? I think it unpardonable for the therapist to sit silently during the first or second interview and wait for the patient to say something. This early in the relationship, the patient does not know the sort of game he is expected to play. Courtesy and tact as well as analytic principles require that the therapist discover why the patient cannot proceed beyond stating the initial complaint.

At first, some further explanation of the nature of the therapeutic situation may be in order. The patient may be laboring under certain misapprehensions—for example, that he has to say everything that comes into his mind or that he must not withhold any information from the therapist—and may be resisting such coercion. Or he may not know what the therapist wants to hear about and may therefore be waiting for more specific guidance. In this sort of situation, I explain to the patient that I can work only on the basis of information he provides, that he may tell me anything he considers important, that he need not tell me anything that he does not want to disclose, and that the relationship between us is absolutely confidential.

This sort of clarification (naturally, not all of this need be said at once) often uncorks the silence. Should it fail to do so, the patient may be asked why he finds it difficult to express himself. Under no circumstances, however, should the therapist be coerced by the patient's silence or by his request that the therapist ask him questions. If the therapist is to practice autonomous psychotherapy, he must have a patient who is able and willing to be self-expressive—within the limits the patient may choose. This demand on the patient must not only be explained verbally, but must be acted on from the start. If the therapist begins, in the first hour, by asking the patient to tell him about his mother, his childhood, or what not—and so *directs* him to behave in a certain way—the patient may expect the therapist to continue such directive behavior. Hence, the therapist must, at the earliest possible moment, indicate that he expects the patient to assume responsibility for communicating or not communicating with the therapist.

If the patient is interested in self-exploration and the therapist is skillful, tactful, and not defensive about the nature and value of what he is doing, a meaningful dialogue between them will develop. In the course of this, the patient will progressively disclose himself, and the therapist will correspondingly disclose the method of his psychotherapeutic effort. To the extent that either party defaults on his contribution to this enterprise, therapy will falter. To repeat, I believe that the therapist's primary responsibility—beyond listening attentively, intelligently, and imaginatively to what the patient tells him—is to apprise the patient of the therapist's position in the situation. This can be and, indeed, must be done in varying ways. Only a few examples can be mentioned here.

For example, in discussing his wife, the patient may suggest that the therapist talk to her. One cannot overlook such a comment. Nor can one counter it, like a comic-strip analyst, by saying inanely: "Why would you like me to do that?" The patient's suggestion calls for a simple but clear explanation of the therapist's policy of not communicating with anyone but the patient. Only in this way can it become a living reality to the patient (and to the analyst, too, for that matter) that the therapy he is about to engage in is for *him,* not for someone else. If the patient wishes to involve his wife in his therapy, he is free to do so, of course; but he is not free to involve his analyst with her.

Issues that often become difficult problems in therapy can be avoided or at least unraveled if the therapist has a clear conception of the therapeutic game acceptable to him. He must make the rules of this game clear to his client and must abide by them himself. A college student, for example, may seek therapy because of learning difficulties and conflicts over choice of a career. At the end of the first hour, he casually remarks that he has not maintained an adequate average and was asked by the dean of men either to leave school or get some therapy. "Will you please call the school and tell them I am in treatment with you?", he asks. If the therapist calls the school, his role as analyst is, in my opinion, finished. For, by consenting, the therapist allows the patient to involve him in the arrangement with the school administration that lets the patient continue in school without performing adequately. In addition, the therapist sets a precedent for participating in the patient's extra-analytic life. If the analyst acts in this fashion once, why not again?

There are, of course, many ways to handle such a situation, but only one that is autonomous and psychoanalytic. The simplest course of action is to comply with the patient's request; this may be especially tempting to the economically insecure therapist, who may sense that, unless he does so, he will lose the patient. Another solution is to interpret to the patient that he is trying to "use" therapy as a substitute for meeting academic standards and yet let him do it. This pseudoanalytic double-talk reassures the therapist; having cleared his conscience with the interpretation, he feels free to communicate with the school authorities. The analyst must repudiate such solutions of the problem. He cannot act collusively; he must act autonomously. This means that he must in no way interfere with the patient's free use of the therapy relationship. What the patient does with it is his concern. At the same time, the therapist must not allow himself to participate in the patient's extra-analytic life.

Accordingly, he must explain to the patient that the agreement to use therapy as a school requirement was arranged by the student and the school authorities, not by the analyst; indeed, he cannot agree to it and will play no part in it. What happens next? If the school authorities acted in good faith and wanted only to secure psychotherapy for the student, they will probably accept his assurance that he has done so or, if they wish proof, the therapist's monthly statement or the patient's canceled check. However, if this does not satisfy the school authorities and they insist on communicating with the therapist about the student's "progress" in therapy, then, once again, the conditions for analysis no longer exist. It is better to find this out early than late.

I wish to emphasize, once again, that, in this sort of situation, the autonomous therapist does not decide that he cannot analyze the patient. To do so would be inappropriate and incorrect. Assuming that the patient is interested in analysis and is otherwise acceptable to the analyst, the therapist's task is to refuse to be drawn into the agreement between the student and the school. Anything more would be an infringement of the patient's freedom of choice. For example, the student may decide to continue with the analysis and let the school authorities decide whether they permit him to continue in school. This means that the patient must be allowed complete freedom in his negotiations with the school authorities. Hence, the analyst cannot interpret as unacceptable "acting-out" the student's use of analysis as an excuse from academic performance, although he must, of course, show the student the kind of game it is. Conversely, the student must be made aware of the analyst's intention to remain uninvolved. If the student believes that he cannot deal with the school single-handed, that he needs an ally who will negotiate for him, then he is either not a fit subject for analysis (at this particular time) or his involvement with the school must be further clarified before analysis can begin.

Before the first interview is terminated, the therapist must raise two subjects, if the client has not already done so. One is the fee; the other, the time and frequency of further appointments.

The financial arrangement between therapist and client must be clearly understood and strictly followed. I discuss the fee with the patient and explain my practice of rendering a statement at the end of each month. Once the fee is set, it should not be changed; it is part of the binding contract between therapist and patient.

Should the therapist have reason to believe that the patient can ill afford the cost of therapy, he should discuss this question with the patient. I do not accept clients for whom the cost of analysis is a significant economic hardship. Strained financial circumstances do not provide a suitable psychological atmosphere for this kind of therapeutic work. Indeed, the situation breeds justified antagonism toward the therapist and is likely to engender a masochistic posture in the analysand.

It may be clear at the end of the first interview that the patient is eager to pursue a further clarification of his situation with the therapist, or it may become evident only after several exploratory interviews. At this point, the therapist must decide whether he wishes to work with the patient, for, the more sessions the therapist has with the patient, the more obligated he is, in my opinion, to continue seeing the patient. I have not found this to be much of a problem, for I can maintain a good therapeutic interest in most persons who want to work with me. Perhaps there is a sort of natural selection during the first few interviews which results in the merging into a single category of two groups of persons: those whom I would prefer not to treat and those who would prefer not to be treated by me. In any case, if the therapist has reason to believe that he does not wish to treat a particular person, he should avoid delving deeply into his life story. The sooner such a client is discharged or referred to a colleague, the better it is.

If both patient and therapist wish to continue, how often should they meet to provide the continuity and depth necessary for analysis? A desirable minimum is three sessions per week;

four are preferable. Nowadays, I rarely see patients five or more times a week, although I did in the past. Occasionally I see a patient twice a week.

The ideal frequency and spacing of appointments will depend on both the patient and the analyst. Young and inexperienced therapists should see their patients relatively often; otherwise they will not be able to understand them. Experienced and skillful therapists, on the other hand, may be able to do analytic work with slightly more discontinuous sessions. In any case, I regard the absolute minimum as two hours per week; this arrangement works only if the therapist is skillful and the patient well equipped and motivated for self-exploration. However, some therapists find three appointments a week generally insufficient, and even the most astute analyst may need more exposure to some patients who are difficult to understand.

With these principles in mind, the therapist may suggest to the patient that they embark on a trial period for a certain number of sessions per week at a certain fee per session. Each session should last fifty minutes. Attempts to use shorter sessions are deplorable. If the patient agrees to this proposal, the trial period begins.

11

The Trial Period

WHY IS A TRIAL PERIOD NECESSARY?

It is difficult for a therapist to form an adequate impression of a patient's personality in one or two interviews. Faced with this problem, many therapists rely on technical procedures to provide them with additional "diagnostic" information; the patient is subjected to intensive questioning about his history, to "stress interviews" and "trial interpretations," to demands for his dreams and fantasies, and, last but not least, to psychological tests (particularly the Rorschach and the Thematic Apperception Test).

None of these measures are compatible with the practice of autonomous psychotherapy, for their aim is to make the patient disclose more information about himself than he chooses. Moreover, such methods of psychological entrapment are neither reliable nor very effective. And, if they accomplish their purpose, they are worse than useless for the analyst because they create precisely that type of psychological relationship between client and therapist that both must persistently try to avoid.

In the first interview or two, neither therapist nor patient can decide whether to proceed with therapy. However, it is desirable that the patient have a chance to know what therapy is like. Therefore, it is best for patient and therapist to begin with an honest recognition of the need to know each other better before they can decide on their future relationship. If they want to continue after the first few interviews, the next phase should accordingly be defined as a trial period.

During the trial period, the therapist can try out the patient, and the patient, the therapist. For the therapist, these sessions provide an opportunity to become better acquainted with the patient—his history, his present situation, his aspirations, and so forth; for the patient, they provide an opportunity to become familiar with the analyst's therapeutic style—what he does and does not do, when he speaks and when he remains silent, what he expects and demands, and so forth. There is no shortcut to this process. No Rorschach protocol can properly introduce a patient to an analyst, nor can a professional recommendation of the therapist properly introduce him to a patient. In discussing the trial period, I usually tell the patient that its aim is, not only to give each of us a chance to observe the other, but to help him understand through this sample experience what he is undertaking.

The trial period serves another function as well. It provides an opportunity for negotiating and defining the therapeutic contract. (This term, "therapeutic contract," refers to the rules by which therapist and patient propose to play the "game of therapy.") Initially, the patient does not know the rules of the analytic game. The therapist does not know whether the patient is capable of playing by these rules and, if capable, whether he is interested in playing. The best way for the therapist to explain the rules of the game and for the patient to understand them before deciding to participate in the game is for the two to engage in a trial game. This is the basic aim of the trial period.

To be sure, the therapist impresses the rules of the analytic game, informally and indirectly, on the patient from the moment they first make contact, for example, by insisting that the patient himself make the first appointment. During the trial period, the rules are made increasingly explicit; they also constitute a subject for discussion and, within certain limits, for negotiation between the two parties. Let us review the principal rules that must be discussed and clarified before patient and therapist can begin the contractual phase of the treatment.

A Preliminary Definition of the Analytic Game

At the beginning of the trial period, the patient may be aware of only two rules: that he must pay a certain fee and that the analyst will avoid instructing him on how to behave, either in the therapeutic situation or outside of it. Even some aspects of these two conditions may not be fully clarified. Almost everything else about therapy is likely to be either unknown or uncertain to the patient.

Frequency of Sessions

Early in the trial period or sometimes even before it, analyst and patient must discuss the frequency of the sessions. I like to begin by scheduling three or four sessions a week. The number that I suggest for now (as against later, before beginning the contractual phase) depends on both our schedules and sometimes also on the patient's financial situation. I explain to the patient that these considerations play a role in this decision and, if necessary, that there is a need for continuity in the treatment. Finally, I often mention that we can reconsider the issue of the frequency of sessions as we proceed with the trial period.

The Couch

Methodologically, the trial period differs from later phases of the treatment in only one important way: no binding contract between patient and therapist has been established. It is necessary, therefore, to consider whether the patient should sit up or lie down. In my office, the patient uses a couch with a back-rest, equally comfortable for sitting and lying. I invite the patient to assume whichever position he prefers. If the patient asks which position I prefer, I tell him that it makes little difference to me, but, that, if it does not matter to him, I prefer his lying down. I believe that, if the therapist only recommends but does not *insist* on either position, the therapeutic situation remains sufficiently free. However, the therapist's belief that analysis can be carried out only when the patient reclines may be a source of serious difficulties.

Free Association and the Fundamental Rule

Freud required that the patient "freely associate," that is, not consciously censor his thoughts, and that he frankly report his "free associations" to the analyst. I believe that this rule is too coercive; it gives the patient the impression that he *must* do something, which, as I define the rules of the game, he need not. Specifically, Freud required "complete candor" from the analysand. In return, he promised him "the strictest discretion." This pact, he said, constitutes the analytic situation.*

Though having the same aim as Freud, I prefer to proceed in a slightly different fashion. I explain to the patient (if he does not already know it) that I can work only with the information he supplies. I encourage him to speak about anything he wishes; I may also indicate that he is free to withhold information, but I add that I can know only what he tells me. For my part, I promise complete confidentiality.

This arrangement, rather than requiring the patient to "free-associate" or to reveal himself as fully as possible, defines the situation in more functional terms. The analysand becomes familiar with the procedure and is made responsible for what he communicates.

* *An Outline of Psychoanalysis* [1938] (New York: Norton, 1940), p. 63.

Dreams

Unless the patient broaches the subject, I do not mention dreams early in the trial period. Although I think that dreams are meaningful communications and make use of them in therapy, I do not believe that they are the royal road to the unconscious. If the analyst seriously believes that they are, he is likely to encourage the patient to report dreams; this distorts the analytic procedure. In terms of psychoanalytic method, however, this exemplifies a problem more general than the issue of dreams.

I maintain that the analyst must not consider any particular topic—dreams, sexuality, childhood events, current problems, transference, or what not—more important or more interesting than any other. Such ranking of subjects imposes formal structure on the analytic situation and thus deprives the patient of the freedom to define the situation for himself. It also reflects the analyst's theoretical bias toward therapy. At the same time, it serves to reinforce that bias, as self-fulfilling prophecies do. By inviting the patient to communicate on a particular subject (e.g., sexuality) or in terms of a particular idiom (e.g., dreams, symptoms), the analyst reconfirms his prejudice about the patient's difficulties and the personality change necessary to correct it.

The analyst may and, indeed, should have only two preferences about the patient's conduct. He should prefer verbal communication to nonverbal and direct communication to indirect. No other preferences would be compatible with the ethic of autonomy.

Medical Procedures

Most patients who consult me do not feel physically ill or think that they need medical help, nor do I have reason to believe otherwise. They rarely expect me to examine them physically or to participate in any other way in their health care.

Let us assume, however, that the patient's physical health is in doubt and that he expects some sort of medical help from the therapist. What should the analyst do? He should explain that, although a physician (if he is), he does no work ordinarily considered medical. Not only does this take care of the issue of physical examination, but also the issues of drugs and of all other organic therapies. Thus the therapist defines his work with the patient as solely psychological or educational. If necessary, the therapist may specify that, as analyst, he listens and talks, tries to clarify problems and situations, discusses alternative courses of action and other types of choice, and tries to decode concealed messages. For emphasis, he may add that he does *nothing else*. It is irrelevant whether the therapist is qualified to help the patient in other ways, for example, by prescribing sedatives or giving advice. The therapist eschews other interventions, not because he is unable to perform them adequately, but because they distract from the task which the analyst and the analysand have set for themselves.

Communication with Third Parties

I maintain a strict policy: no involvement with anyone but the patient. Once the matter has been discussed, I expect the patient to discourage other people from communicating with me about him or his analysis. At the same time, because I do not place any restrictions on the patient, he is free to put the analysis to whatever use he pleases. He may brag about it or hide it; he may try to use it to his advantage at school or work, or his career may suffer because of it; he may use the analyst's monthly statement as evidence in court or income-tax proceedings or may choose not to; and so forth.

Let us consider a typical example. The analysand may request letters or statements for draft boards, schools, and various agencies. It is often said that the therapist should be careful in such cases lest he harm his patient; he should release information only with the patient's understanding and consent. But to proceed in this way is to miss the point of analysis altogether.

In autonomous therapy, it does not really matter whether, by communicating with third parties, the analyst "helps" or "harms" the patient. (The distinction is empty partly because it is often impossible to know in advance the actual consequence of such actions.) Indeed, in proportion as the patient succeeds in securing extra-analytic help from the analyst, he succeeds in making the analysis a noxious, rather than therapeutic, influence on him. For example, the patient is a failing student for whom, because he is "in therapy" and is "doing well," the analyst recommends leniency to the school authorities. By doing this, the therapist elevates himself to a power position he ought not to have and reduces the patient to that heteronomous and irresponsible position from which the analysis is supposed to rescue him.

This is not to say that the therapist should be cold and disinterested about such issues. First of all, they are grist for the analytic mill. Second, the analyst must, as always, be helpful in discussing the patient's aspirations and the methods by which he plans to pursue them. While standing firm in his determination to maintain analytic autonomy, the therapist should be as helpful as he can to liberate the patient and enable him to pursue his ends by *any* method he chooses. Here is an example. Although the analyst would not perform an abortion on a patient who desires one, he must be as free in discussing the "reality situation" concerning abortions, both in his own country and abroad, as he is about the "reality situation" of, say, the patient's job. The same sort of consideration applies to everything the patient wants to do outside the analysis and for which he asks the analyst's help.

Mental Hospitalization and Suicide

Some patients go through a long analysis and never mention committing suicide. Others relate suicidal thoughts or complain of fears that they may kill themselves early in therapy. Similarly, some patients may never raise the issue of mental hospitalization, whereas others may discuss it during the first meeting with the therapist. Indeed, some patients who consult the analyst may have been previously hospitalized; others may have attempted suicide. I combine these two phenomena here because the threat of suicide is often a reason for recommending psychiatric hospitalization to a patient (or, if he refuses, for committing him) and also because the autonomous therapist's position on these two problems is identical.

During the trial period, if the patient does not raise the question of mental hospitalization and I have no reason to believe that it may become an issue later, I do not mention it either. But, as I have emphasized, I do everything I can to explain to the patient that I promise only to analyze him and that all contacts will take place in my office.

Should the question of the patient needing mental hospitalization arise early in therapy, the analyst must explain to the patient that he does not practice hospital psychiatry. If the patient believes that he requires confinement in a hospital, for his own protection or for that of others, he has to seek it, like everything else nonanalytic, from someone other than the analyst. The analyst may offer to recommend hospital facilities, as he might recommend an internist or surgeon to a patient who requests such information, but he ought to go no further. This stand is necessary; it protects the integrity of the analytic situation and assures the patient that the analyst has renounced the standard psychiatric role which permits him to hospitalize "mental patients" with or without their consent.

In brief, the analyst must relinquish playing the mental-hospital game for good, and the analysand must be certain of this. It is curious how easily analysts have accepted the rule that they must not examine their patients physically. But they have not accepted the rule that they must not participate in their mental hospitalization either. Thus, the analyst must not only relinquish the customary role of physician, but also that of psychiatrist.

As with physical examinations or drugs, the patient must be free to make his own decisions about mental hospitalization; at the same time, as long as the patient complies with the rules of the analytic game, the analyst must be willing to analyze him.

The analyst's stand on the threat of suicide is the same; he cannot allow it to become a ground for modifying the contract. This understanding benefits both patient and therapist. For some people, self-destruction is more of a possibility than for others. The analyst's task is to analyze this craving or fear as he would any other. For the analyst to act on the danger of the patient's suicide—other than perhaps to discuss, among other possible courses of action, the patient's seeking hospitalization—is to relinquish the analytic mandate and to "act out." Indeed, only if the patient is deeply convinced that the analyst respects his autonomy, including his right to take his own life, can he engage effectively in the analytic exploration and mastery of his ideas about suicide. With such understanding between patient and therapist, the analysand's communications about suicide remain the language of self-destruction which it is the analyst's task to analyze; without it, the analysand's communications become coercive messages intended to influence the therapist's conduct.

How Does the Trial Period End?

The duration of the trial period varies. It depends,. first, on the patient, on what sort of problem he brings to the therapist and on what kind of solution he seeks for it. Second, it depends on the therapist, on when he feels ready to undertake autonomous psychotherapy with the patient. In my experience, the trial period may be as short as a week or two or may extend over many months and never be converted into another kind of arrangement.

The trial period tends to be shortest with those patients who are both well informed about analytic matters and who want to be analyzed. Many of my patients—as is also true of analytic patients generally—are professional men and women. Some have had previous experience with psychotherapy. They learn rapidly what I expect of them. In such cases, I can often decide in a half-dozen sessions or less whether I can work with the patient. If I have no reason to believe that the patient cannot adhere to the rules of the analytic game and we can agree on the fee and a mutually convenient schedule of appointments, then I almost always accept the patient for treatment.

At the other extreme, the trial period may run into several months. For example, the patient may complain of problems that are so complex or so vague that it requires a great deal of work to clarify why he came and what he wants; or he may have had previous experience with analysis or psychotherapy and may be hesitant about embarking on another period of therapy; or he may be a student poised between continuing in school and dropping out or between staying in the city where the analyst lives and transferring to a school elsewhere. In these and similar situations, the patient usually prefers to continue therapy over an extended period, but on a somewhat tentative basis.

It is undesirable to bring pressure on such persons either to "enter analysis" (that is, to make a commitment to regular appointments over many months) or to drop out. Instead, I accept the patient's terms, if he can accept mine. Accordingly, what ensues is an extended trial period. Appointments are scheduled for only one week at a time. Instead of promising the patient that I will be available to him as long as he wants to come, I commit myself only to seeing him until his problem is clarified, he is referred to another therapist, we convert to a regular therapeutic arrangement, or, finally, until he chooses to stop. In some cases, the entire course of the therapy consists of such a "trial period"; when it is over, the patient decides that this was all he needed or wanted.

Sometimes the patient who seems to be in a chaotic situation and not at all ready to settle down to analytic routine wants to end the trial period and begin "the regular analysis." This is usually due to the patient's fear that the therapist may discontinue therapy and thus "reject" him; the patient may try to protect himself against this threat by making the sort of promises he thinks the therapist expects of him. I refuse to comply with such a request and explain to the patient my reason for doing so. I may point to major areas in the patient's life that I do not understand or to problems which promise to interfere with the analysis. In some of these cases, we go on to analysis. In others, a further period of therapy makes it clear that the patient is actually unwilling to abide by the rules of analysis; the patient had really expected the therapist to relax his expectations, and, when he realizes that the therapist will not do so, he stops.

It may also happen that the patient, fearful of being abandoned by the therapist, uses the tentativeness of the trial period for his own emotional needs. This contingency, of course, requires analysis; the same situation would have arisen if patient and therapist had agreed to proceed with intensive therapy earlier. There are many other expectations, needs, and problems that patients and therapists bring to the therapeutic situation that color the meaning of the trial period for each. There is no substitute for trying to understand as much as possible about what happens in therapy and for stating it clearly. The patient must be enlisted in this venture, for without him it cannot succeed.

12

The Contractual Phase:

I. Implementing the Contract

THE MAIN DIFFERENCE BETWEEN the trial period and the contractual phase of therapy lies in the kind of commitment the analyst makes to the patient. In the former, his commitment is provisional and qualified; in the latter, it is enduring and unqualified. Before entering the contractual phase, analyst and analysand must come to an understanding about the sort of commitment the therapist is preparing to make; he is offering the patient his services as analyst for as long as the patient wants them and is willing to comply with his obligations to the analyst.

Fulfillment of the analytic contract depends largely on whether the analyst takes the necessary steps to implement it. It is not enough for the analyst to announce a contract; when the time comes, he must act. It is not enough to predict the sort of moves one will make in a game; at the proper moment, one must make the move. Not only words, but moves, too, provide information; in analysis, both types of information are exchanged by the participants. If the analyst makes all the correct interpretations

178

to the patient, but does not also support them with the correct moves, his analytic efforts will be vitiated.

IMPLEMENTING THE ANALYTIC CONTRACT

The moves by which the therapist defines the game were indicated in the discussion of the trial period. In the contractual phase, the therapist will be called upon to further define and interpret many of the game rules. The only new rule that comes into effect at this time (but one that will have been discussed during the trial period) is the therapist's promise to continue treatment until the patient wishes to terminate it and its corollary, his refusal to make the decision to terminate. During the contractual phase, the patient is likely to test this rule in various ways. Its ultimate implication, however—namely, that the patient himself must decide when to end treatment—comes into focus only during the terminal period.

Although it has significance in its own right, the main purpose of the contract is to create a situation suitable for psychoanalytic learning. Thus, a great deal of therapeutic work during the contractual phase is in analyzing the patient's problems in more or less traditional ways. I shall not say much about this aspect of analytic technique. For hints about the sorts of thing to look for and do and about certain other aspects of analysis (for example, defenses, transference, and so forth), the reader is referred to the classic writings of Fenichel, Freud, Glover, and the other analytic masters.

We may proceed, then, to a further consideration of the contractual phase of autonomous psychotherapy, paying special attention to the measures used to implement the contract.

The Scheduling of Appointments

The analyst has no product to sell; he cannot cure an illness, prescribe a drug to allay the patient's anxiety, or provide a medical excuse for a patient's obligation. He can contract only for the sale of *time* and *services*.

It is implicit in the contract and must often be made explicit that the services are promised for delivery in a certain fashion. In other words, the therapist must be punctual; he must begin and end the sessions in accordance with the prearranged agreement. Since analysts generally adhere to this rule, I shall not dwell on it. However, many therapists also expect their patients to be punctual. In my opinion, this illustrates a basic misunderstanding of the relationship between analyst and analysand.

Therapist and patient do not follow the same rules. Their roles are complementary, not interchangeable. The two are equal in that each must respect the autonomy of the other and that power is distributed (nearly) equally between them. In terms of rule-following, however, the relation between analyst and analysand is a cooperative one, comparable to the relation between doubles partners in tennis. For the duration of a game, one player serves, the other is at the net; though both play tennis, each plays by a somewhat different set of rules.

In autonomous psychotherapy, most of the restrictions are placed on the analyst; the patient has great freedom of action. For example, he is under no obligation to be punctual for his appointments with the therapist. He must be punctual only in paying his bill. Let us remember that the patient approaches the analyst wishing to purchase his services. We may assume, therefore, that he has an incentive to accept delivery of the merchandise he wishes to buy. Indeed, most patients are punctual. However, they have a right not to be. When they are habitually late, the analyst's task is to seek the reasons for this behavior and, if he understands it, to interpret it. Were the analyst to punish the patient for being late or to influence him to be more punctual, he would be stepping out of his role as analyst.

Cancellation of appointments creates a similar problem. From time to time, the analyst, as well as the patient, will find it necessary to cancel appointments. In general, the reasons will be professional interests or duties, personal needs or plans, or illness. Analysts have traditionally followed a one-sided policy; they could cancel, but the patient could not (or, if he did, he had to pay for his appointment). If this rule is followed, it places a heavy and quite unnecessary burden on the analytic relationship. The rule is clearly discriminatory against the patient. It violates the principles of the analytic contract. The analyst promises to deliver a service to the patient regularly and punctually; yet, to fulfill his personal needs, he retains the privilege of interrupting delivery. If the therapist may have this privilege (and, of course, he should), why not the patient also?

The usual explanation for having the patient pay for canceled appointments (regardless of the cause) is that the analyst has leased an hour of his time and that the patient is responsible for it. But this argument is contradicted by the analyst's behavior; he says that he has leased an hour, but remains free to absent himself from the appointment. Were he *really* leasing "time," he would be obliged to compensate the patient. This is common practice in commercial life; for example, a contractor is responsible for monetary damages for the delayed completion of a building. The analyst who goes to Europe for a two-month vacation delays "delivery" on his patient's analysis. I am not suggesting that he should not do this, but I am pointing out that he does it without compensating the patient for the inconvenience.

Accordingly, if the therapist wishes to make the relationship between him and his patient as egalitarian as possible, he must give the the patient the same privileges for cancellation as he himself enjoys. Thus, the patient must be allowed to cancel because he wants to attend a professional meeting or go to Europe without having to pay for the canceled appointments. (This is less likely to be a problem for the therapist who earns a good income than for the one who does not.)

A brief remark about another kind of cancellation is pertinent here. The analytic contract involves the following exchange: the analyst sells his services; the patient buys these services, and (this is the point here) must take delivery of them in the analyst's office. What happens if the patient alters his situation (or his situation becomes altered through no "fault" or active intervention on his part) so that he cannot visit the analyst's office? This may occur, for example, if the patient is imprisoned for crime, hospitalized for psychosis, or incapacitated (for more than a few days) by illness. In such circumstances, the analyst's responsibility toward the patient ceases, at least for this period. (The analyst cannot go to the patient and deliver his services, say, in the patient's home or in a hospital.)

Such an interruption may be handled in one of two ways, depending on the patient's preferences and the prior agreement which analyst and analysand have made about this contingency. If the patient wishes to resume his visits to the analyst as soon as he can do so, he must pay for his nonattendance. On the other hand, if he prefers not to pay for unkept "visits" over what may be an extended period, he may elect not paying but having to wait, not only until he is ready to visit the analyst again, but until the analyst's normal schedule permits resuming the relationship. The analyst must, of course, take the patient back and not penalize him for the interruption. Only in this way can the analysand's attendance at the analyst's office be made an obligation and a responsibility which the patient owes to himself, not to the analyst; the therapist neither rewards nor punishes him for failure to meet it.

In my practice, I give patients the same privileges to cancel as I take for myself. Nonattendance rarely becomes a problem. However, sometimes, especially with hypochondriacal patients, it does; I then give the patient a choice between paying for appointments canceled for "illness" and discontinuing therapy.

Entanglements in Nonanalytic Procedures

The therapist's autonomy as analyst and the patient's as analysand may be undermined at any point during the treatment by a variety of needs which either participant may wish to satisfy. The principal danger to a fully contractual and mutually autonomous relationship lies in the need of each to coerce the other. This risk is partly psychological, stemming from the aspirations of the two parties to the contract, and partly situational, deriving from the social expectancies built into the roles of sufferer and helper. Thus, as therapist, the analyst may readily assume a superior position; he must therefore constantly guard against this. The patient, on the other hand, may readily assume an inferior position and resort to the main strength of a position of weakness, that is, using suffering to coerce his partner. The therapist must, therefore, also guard against the patient's strategy of gaining the upper hand by the paradoxical maneuver of seizing on what appears to be an inferior role.

Giving advice and prescribing drugs are frequent causes of imbalance in the analytic relationship. In these ways, the therapist communicates to the client his readiness to assume some measure of *control* of the patient's impulses, needs, or problems. If he does so, who will decide the extent of the control the therapist ought to assume? And how will it be decided?

These questions cannot be answered. In practice, the patient will often tempt the psychiatrist to assume ever more control of him. He will do this by acting as though he were progressively losing self-control. The more advice the psychiatrist gives and the more drugs he prescribes, the more the patient will seem to deteriorate; he will become increasingly depressed and "helpless" and need more and more sedatives. Correspondingly, the pressure on the psychiatrist to "do something" will mount. Before long, the therapist will begin to worry that the patient may commit suicide. He may now try to increase his control over the patient by hospitalizing him, treating him with electroshock, and so forth. In this vicious cycle, the patient may be able to prove that he is his own master only by killing himself. Of course, once the therapist starts down this road, he has given up, or should have given up, all hope of analyzing his patient.

The competent analyst should not need to do such things. He should limit himself to being an analyst. Perhaps it is appropriate here to comment on why the therapist may find the analytic posture difficult to maintain.

If the patient can be defined as dependent, helpless, and sick, the therapist is justified in assuming a measure of control of him. Since such persons require protection, the role of "protector" becomes legitimized. On the other hand, if the therapist considers the patient autonomous and self-responsible, protection is not legitimate. If such a person is nevertheless "protected," we may rightly speak of degradation, exploitation, and oppression. An example of this is the relationship between segregationists and Negroes.

It is evident why providing protection is attractive to the protector; it gives him control of the relationship. Herein lies the crux of the problem for therapists who find the posture of autonomy difficult; by relinquishing the "duty" to protect the patient, they must also relinquish the "privilege" of controlling him. The autonomous therapist has virtually no control of his patient; hence he may fear losing him. It follows, then, that, in proportion as the therapist is afraid of object loss, he will seek a heteronomous type of relationship with his patients. Psychotherapists often need their patients more than patients need their psychotherapists (not only economically, but psychologically as well). Thus, to overcome one of the limits on the practice of autonomous psychotherapy, the therapist must be largely free of the fear of losing his patient and, hence, of the wish to control him.

Another kind of nonanalytic entanglement that the therapist must avoid is communicating about the patient with third parties. Quite erroneously, the utility of this practice is often considered to consist in the protection of the patient's confidences. To be sure, these need absolute protection; and, if the analyst does not discuss the patient with others, the patient's confidences are, *ipso facto,* perfectly protected. This is as it should be. However, restricting the analyst's relationship to his patient alone serves another purpose as well. To see this clearly, let us consider a contingency by no means infrequent in psychotherapy.

Let us suppose that the patient wants to release the therapist from the obligation of keeping his communications confidential and, further, that he requests the therapist to communicate with others, for example, to give a diagnosis to the dean of a college or to the personnel director of a business firm. What should the analyst do?

I need not dwell on the fact that the analyst does not play an ordinary medical game. The "material" that the analysand communicates to the analyst is not like the blood specimen which the medical patient gives to his physician. In the latter case, the patient "owns" the blood and hence also the information which the doctor may extract from it. Accordingly, the patient can instruct the physician to transmit this information to third parties, and, in the ordinary course of events, the doctor will do so. He has no reason not to.

It is foolish, however, to try to follow the same rules in analysis, for there is nothing the analyst could communicate to others which the patient does not also know or is not entitled to know. Since the purpose of analysis is to maximize the patient's autonomy, the analyst has no more reason to inform a third party of the patient's "diagnosis" than to tell the patient's wife that her husband hates her or the patient's stockbroker that his client wants to buy a hundred shares of General Motors at 92. Whatever the patient wants the various people in his life to know, *he* can tell them; in fact, he must tell them, for the analyst will not do so for him. Were the analyst to play this sort or role, he would participate actively in the patient's extra-analytic life and so vitiate the entire analytic effort.

"Frustrating" and "Satisfying" the Patient

The problem of how much the analyst should satisfy or frustrate the patient has long plagued psychoanalysis. Freud's views on this have not helped matters. Confronted with phobic and obsessional patients who, despite intensive analytic work, were unwilling to relinquish their symptoms, Freud suggested that the therapist adopt certain kinds of "activity" to bring pressure on the patient to change. The "fundamental principle" that he proposed was: "Analytic treatment should be carried through, as far as is possible, under privation—in a state of abstinence."°

This dictum has proved to be a rich source of confusion. To be sure, by "abstinence," Freud did not mean sexual abstinence. Ferenczi and others, however, did advise patients not to masturbate or have sexual intercourse. But Freud's suggestions in regard to abstinence were only slightly less unfortunate:

> Cruel though it may sound, we must see to it that the patient's suffering, to a degree that is in some way or other effective, does not come to an end prematurely. . . . As far as his relations with the physician are concerned, the patient must be left with unfulfilled wishes in abundance. It is expedient to deny him precisely those satisfactions which he desires most intensely and expresses most importunely.†

Here we see Freud advocating manipulating and coercing the patient, ostensibly in the interests of analysis. This is absurd. Such maneuvers are antianalytic and have no place in autonomous psychotherapy. The problems that made Freud resort to such "active" interventions are readily clarified by considering psychoanalysis a contractual relationship; it is appropriate to say something about them here.

I believe that Freud formulated the rule of abstinence to counteract the therapist's "natural" tendency to comfort the patient. Thus, he felt it necessary to emphasize that the analyst should not comply with the patient's wishes *if* they obstruct the work of analysis. For example, should the patient long for the therapist's affection, the analyst should not give it merely to make her "feel better." The aim of therapy is not to achieve "happiness" or even "well-being," but to learn about one's self and develop personal autonomy. To me, the rule of abstinence means just this, and nothing more recondite.

° "Lines of Advance in Psycho-Analytic Therapy" [1919], *The Standard Edition of the Complete Psychological Works of Sigmund Freud,* XVII (London: Hogarth Press, 1955), 162.

† *Ibid.,* pp. 163–164.

However, for a number of reasons which need not concern us here, the idea became popular in psychoanalysis that the proper psychological condition for a patient undergoing analysis was a state of frustration. Thus, many analysts believe that patients *ought* to feel anxious, make a financial sacrifice for the treatment, and so forth because, if they do not, the analysis will fail to be effective. In my opinion, this view is completely false.* The analyst has no more right to "frustrate" his patient than to "gratify" him. Moreover, just what do we mean by "frustration" and "gratification"?

Viewing the analytic relationship as contractual simplifies the matter. The analyst contracts with the patient to do certain things for him. Strictly speaking, then, if the analyst fulfills his contract, he does not "reward" his patient; he merely conducts himself as an honest person who does his job and keeps his promises. Conversely, if the analyst fails to fulfill his contract, he does not "frustrate" his patient (although, to be sure, the patient may *feel* frustrated); he merely conducts himself as a dishonest person who does not do his job and breaks his promises.

Naturally, in practice things are not so simple as this. But let us consider the classic problem that gives rise to the notion of "abstinence" and reformulate it in terms of autonomy and contract. The patient is an attractive young woman whose husband is impotent. She comes to the analyst and falls in love with him. Should he satisfy her sexual cravings? If he does not, she will be "frustrated" and therefore in the proper state of "abstinence" to be analyzed. To me, this is a strange way of looking at the problem.

Although the patient may want to engage in sexual intercourse with the therapist, this is not the kind of activity that the therapist has promised to sell. Hence, this situation requires clarification above all else, and the sooner the better. Perhaps largely because this sort of situation was not adequately clarified in the early days of analysis and also because physicians did occa-

* See Thomas S. Szasz, "The Meaning of Suffering in Therapy," *American Journal of Psychoanalysis,* 21 (1961), 12–17.

sionally engage in sexual activity with their patients, the analytic patient was not wholly unjustified in expecting the therapist to act in a similar fashion. The notion then prevalent that the correct prescription for the disease "hysteria" was *Penis normalis, dosim: repetatur* could not help matters. If this was a "treatment," why should physicians not "administer" it? Let us make no mistake about it; this is no mere play on words. Only in this light can we understand why analysts thought that denying patients certain things is the same as frustrating them. This is, of course, true for persons who are helpless, especially children and the physically disabled. If a baby is hungry, his mother cannot tell him to find some food and feed himself. But is this the appropriate model for the analytic patient?

To return to our hypothetical case of the young hysterical woman who needs "sex," the analyst's task is not to worry about her state of "abstinence," but to find out why, if she wants a lover, she does not look for one outside the analytic situation. Though, of course, *experientially,* this sort of situation is erotic (and, if the patient is attractive, the analyst might be tempted), *theoretically,* it is not specifically sexual in nature. Suppose that the patient's husband lost all his money and that she wanted the analyst to support her. Would he consider refusing financial help to the patient as "frustrating" her? Keeping the contractual nature of autonomous psychotherapy in mind helps both analyst and analysand to avoid confusing and equating adherence to the contract with "frustrating" the patient.

Another aspect of this problem deserves brief mention. From my contacts with young therapists, I have gained the impression that many believe that there is something inherently, mysteriously "good" or "correctly analytic" about refusing to reply to a patient's question simply because he asked it. The therapist might have been on the verge of explaining something, but, in reaction to the patient's direct question, he freezes and remains silent. (This is usually the same therapist who, paradoxically but understandably, will also err in contaminating the analytic situation by doing "too much" for the patient, that is, by doing things not called for in the contract.) Such a therapist is too afraid of being controlled by the patient; he counter-reacts by trying to control the patient.

My point here is that the patient is *entitled* to the sort of help that the analyst has promised to give him. Though some of the patient's questions may remain unanswered—and it is desirable that he understand the need for this—many others deserve a serious answer. In sum, the analyst should have no desire to "frustrate" the patient and hence refuse to answer questions, nor should he have a desire to "gratify" the patient and hence answer questions that ask for reassurance rather than information.

13

The Contractual Phase:

II. Analysis of the

Analytic Situation

THE CONCEPTS OF AUTONOMY AND CONTRACT are crucial to psycho-analysis. It is not surprising, therefore, that the practitioner of this type of therapy will find some of his problems structured in terms of autonomy versus heteronomy, and promise-keeping versus promise-breaking. Many traditional problems of psychiatry and psychotherapy assume a new, more manageable, form when approached from this point of view.

Usually the patient comes to the therapist wanting help for his complaints. He does not come to negotiate a contract. However, this sort of dissonance between buyer and seller is not uncommon. For example, a man may want his life insured; he consults an insurance agent, who explains the contracts offered by various life-insurance companies. The client must decide whether he wants to buy a policy and, if so, what kind.

Likewise, although the patient may come wanting to buy

"therapy," the analyst must first explain what he has to sell. If the patient is uninformed, the analyst must also explain what other kinds of psychiatric therapy are for sale. Unless the patient has a choice among a variety of therapies and therapists, he cannot negotiate effectively with the analyst. If he can obtain help only by submitting to the analyst's conditions, then, in effect, he is coerced by his own need to buy whatever the analyst sells.

Some people approach the therapist in exactly this spirit; they assert that they need therapeutic help that *only* the analyst whom they have consulted can supply; hence, they must submit—and, indeed, will do so willingly—to the analyst's terms. The analyst must not accept this definition of the situation, but must challenge it and try to clarify it. To be sure, the client may sincerely believe that a particular therapist is the only one who can help him. This might occasionally even be true. Nevertheless, it is important to keep in mind that the patient seeking analytic help has choices. The practice of psychoanalysis is possible only in a capitalist society; competitive and pluralistic, such a society offers a variety of therapies for people in quandary. I emphasize this point because, though the patient may feel that only one form of treatment is "right" for him, he has, in fact, chosen it in preference to many others.

Analysis of the Analytic Situation

In large part, the analysis of the analytic situation* is the analysis of the contract. A contractual agreement, by its very nature, may be broken in one of two ways: by underfulfilling or by overfulfilling one's obligations. These two types of contract violation correspond, roughly, to the characterological postures of the person who exploits and the one who allows himself to be exploited. To an extent, the former is typical of the so-called oral-demanding, or greedy, individual or of the sadist, and the latter, of the so-called mature, or generous, person or of the masochist.

* See Chapter 3.

The Person Who Habitually Underfulfills His Contracts

A good example of the person who tries to avoid his contractual obligations is the patient who habitually plays the sick role. He sees nothing in life but his own disabilities, needs, problems, and suffering; he secretly expects that he ought to be and somehow will be rewarded ("helped") for his troubles. This patient says, in effect: "I don't want to negotiate. I just want to have my own way. Why don't you give me what I need so badly?"

Such patients often exhibit, at least initially, hysterical conversion symptoms; or they may suffer from so-called psychosomatic illnesses; or they may be "neurasthenic," complaining of chronic anxiety, fatigue, and depression. At first they seem interested and willing to play the analytic game. But, as the contract is more sharply defined, they rebel against it. Before long, they complain bitterly about the time and money they must invest in the treatment. Next they test the therapist; they cancel appointments and postpone paying their bills. Such patients have often had long, successful careers using such tactics on relatives and sometimes other therapists. They have thus learned that they do not have to keep their promises and can break (or not make any) contracts; their symptoms and suffering are accepted as valid excuses.

In this type of situation, analysis of the contract and of the patient's attitude toward it and, in addition, an uncompromising attitude toward the contract on the part of the therapist are mandatory for effective analytic therapy. If the therapist modifies the contract—for example, by giving the patient sedatives or medical excuses for some purpose or other or by reducing the fee or letting the patient accumulate a debt—then, instead of analyzing the patient's conduct, the therapist will have permitted him to re-enact, in the therapeutic situation, his habitual mode of behavior.

It is as though the patient were saying: "I can't comply with the terms of the contract because I am too sick (or too exhausted, or too pressed for money, and so forth)." The patient thus speaks the language of "I can't," or of excuses. The therapist either accepts this idiom or rejects it. In general, the nonanalytic therapist (especially the so-called supportive therapist) does the former; the analytic therapist, the latter.

The analyst's task is to translate from the language of "I can't" into the language of "I don't want to," or from the language of excuses into the language of responsibility. A great deal of the day-to-day work of analysis consists in making this sort of translation for the patient and of teaching him to make it for himself.

The therapist who fails to challenge the patient's idiom accepts him as an irresponsible person. The psychoanalyst must not do this. He must be able to understand the patient's language, but must refuse to adopt it for the therapeutic encounter. Instead, he must treat the patient as an autonomous, responsible person. This can be achieved only by ascribing responsibility to him and expecting him to assume it. In this respect, therapy is anything but morally neutral. The patient must assume responsibility in order to fulfill his contract with the therapist. If he does not, the contract will be terminated.

This, I might add, is the only way the analyst may coerce the patient. The autonomous therapist cannot and must not directly influence the patient to behave responsibly toward others; that is their problem, not his. This does not mean, of course, that the therapist may not comment on the patient's contract-breaking style of behavior with those close to him.

The Person Who Habitually Overfulfills His Contracts

In contrast to people who habitually cheat or try to get something for nothing, there are those who believe that they must pay a price for everything in life; the more they want something, the higher the price. Here the therapist is confronted by the chronically guilt-ridden person who is afraid of exploiting his partner and being blamed for it. Such a person not only honors his contract, but tends to overfulfill it; he is hyper-responsible. Thus, the patient is oversolicitous of the analyst and his needs; he behaves as though the analyst were weak and the patient strong; he pays his bills promptly and never complains about the cost of the analysis; he offers to do favors for the analyst and tries to bring him gifts; and so forth. Such patients are often willing to contract for an analysis on terms, financial and otherwise, that may be too onerous for them.

As a rule, one or both parents of such people defined their roles in terms of great self-sacrifice for the child. As a result, the child has grown to feel unbearably guilty about the parent's efforts on his behalf and tries to mitigate his guilt by amply "repaying" the parent and, subsequently, anyone who might do something for him. Such persons often become analytic patients because their tendency to overfulfill contracts encourages employers, friends, spouses, and children to exploit them. Sooner or later, they resent this.

These persons, also, speak the language of needs. In contrast to the exploiter who is attuned only to his own needs, the exploitee is attuned to the needs of others, to the exclusion of his own. More precisely, it is vital for such persons to perceive accurately the needs of others and, if possible, to satisfy them. Hence, they overfulfill their contracts and comply too much with the demands of their partners to avoid feeling guilty of defaulting on their obligations.

Both the exploiter and the exploitee present certain problems to the analyst trying to arrange a contractual relationship with the patient. The exploiter opposes the contract because his attitude is: "I am too weak and too helpless to negotiate a contract; you must try to accept me as I am until I grow stronger; then I shall be happy to act more responsibly." Of course, this is the promise that is destined to be broken. Once the therapist accepts it, the analysis is finished.

The exploitee, too, opposes the contract, though he does so more subtly. The unwary therapist may easily miss the import of the patient's behavior and feelings. His attitude may be paraphrased as follows: "I can't negotiate with you because *you* are too weak; though you think we are negotiating, we are not, for I am obliged to accept your terms to avoid hurting you and then feeling responsible for it." Here therapy is threatened by the patient's guilt, masochism, and denial of dependence. If the therapist is unaware of this possibility (which may happen, especially if he needs patients and money), he may enter into a therapeutic arrangement with a patient for whom the required expenditure of time, money, and effort is too much. Thus, what may look like a contract may become a re-enactment of the patient's habitually masochistic life style.

Exchanging Gifts and Favors

Giving and receiving gifts is—in our culture, at least—a fundamental transaction in family life, highly charged with emotional significance. Perhaps better than anything else, the thoughtful gift symbolizes love, affection, and especially gratitude. Accordingly, the "language" of gifts offers the patient a ready medium of communication with the therapist. In medical and nonanalytic psychiatric practice, it is an accepted and "normal" part of the therapeutic relationship for the grateful patient to present his physician with a gift as a token of appreciation for his help. If the patient is wealthy, the gift may be substantial, exceeding by a wide margin the physician's most extravagant fee for the particular service rendered.

Because giving and receiving gifts is so much a normal part of family life and also of many client–expert relationships, the analysand will usually be inclined, some time during therapy or at its conclusion, to present the analyst with a gift. He will also expect to receive favors from him. The therapist, on the other hand, may be tempted to accept gifts from his patient and to bestow favors on him. In this situation, as in so many others, the analyst cannot simply comply with social convention, however convenient this might sometimes be.

Precisely because exchanging gifts and favors possesses great emotional significance for the patient (and possibly also for the therapist) and because it is a conventional activity, such transactions offer the analysand a socially acceptable vehicle for expressing and disguising his transferences to the analyst. The analyst's task is clear; he must analyze such conduct, not engage in it. How can and should the analyst do this?

The analyst must, of course, renounce the wish to receive gifts from his patients or to bestow favors on them. Here, again, an adequate fee plays a role; if the analyst is paid for his services, his wish to "collect" from his patient in extramonetary ways is reduced. The therapist's wish to do favors for the patient is, in many ways, a more complex source of difficulty for analytic work; certainly the analyst who wishes to help his clients through autonomous psychotherapy must master this inclination.

However, even though the analyst might be free of any desire to communicate with the patient through the medium of gifts and favors, the patient may not be. Hence, every analytic therapist must be prepared to deal with this problem tactfully and effectively.

Unlike rules about the fee or the frequency of the sessions, rules about exchanging gifts should not be set down at the beginning of treatment. It would be inappropriate and tactless to do so; at the outset of his relationship with the therapist, the patient is usually occupied with his personal problems and perhaps with his fear of therapy, not with giving presents to the therapist. Hence, if the therapist were to introduce the subject, he would be laying down a prohibition. In some patients, this may serve to stimulate a desire to engage in the prohibited conduct; in others, it may block the subsequent development of a desire to exchange gifts. In either case, the analyst's excessive and premature intrusion into the therapeutic situation would render the analysis of the patient's propensities for communicating through the "language" of gifts more difficult or impossible.

For these reasons, I find it best to deal with the issue of gifts and favors only as it arises in the therapeutic situation. I grant no favors to patients, but do accept small gifts (of slight monetary value) from them—once or sometimes even twice. I proceed in this way because I believe that, in addition to its affectional aspects, giving and receiving gifts is a powerful means of defining the structure of a human encounter. The paradigm situation in which a gift is generously offered and eagerly accepted is the relationship between parent and child. Hence, the giver of a gift tends to feel superior to, or "one up on," its recipient. Thus the saying: "It is easier to give than to receive."

When, in the course of the therapeutic relationship, the patient brings me a small gift, he is acting in a socially appropriate manner; hence, to refuse the gift, even if the refusal is accompanied by explanations, is to put him "one down."

In effect, it is like telling the client that, *because* he is a patient, he is too unimportant to give the therapist a present. However, should the patient already know—as he may, if he is a professional person or otherwise knowledgeable about psychoanalysis—that analysts usually do not accept gifts, then it is appropriate to refuse even the first gift. Also, if the gift is valuable, that is, if it costs more than a fraction of the fee for one session, the analyst must not accept it. Should the analyst accept such a gift, he would be a party to the actual, economic overfulfillment of the patient's analytic contract; he would accept more economic recompense than the fee on which he and the patient had agreed.

Such a posture may entail serious sacrifices on the part of the analyst. In our present moral climate, when everything psychiatrists do is so easily rationalized as serving "therapeutic" goals, such stoic self-discipline is as rare as it is unfashionable. But, since analysts usually do not accept gifts from their patients, why do I emphasize this point so strongly? Because of a compromise that creates the impression that the analyst abstains from this practice, whereas, in fact, he subtly participates in it. I refer to those instances in which, at the conclusion of his therapy, a wealthy analysand gives a substantial sum of money to support his analyst's research, institute, or organization. Although the money is not given directly to the therapist nor during the therapy, it is nevertheless given to the analyst and is in reality a part of the analytic relationship.

Such bequests are, of course, similar to those which affluent expatients often make to hospitals and research organizations. However, a gift of this type by a former analytic patient cannot be compared to one by a former medical patient. Rather, it must be compared to what would correspond to it in the analyst's own conduct. What would this be? It would consist in the analyst "donating" to the patient the fee for the last several months of therapy, that is, treating the patient gratis during the terminal period or perhaps giving him a large sum of money after termination. This would generally be considered a grievous violation of the analytic relationship. I contend that accepting the financial largess of exanalysands is a similar violation of the analytic relationship.

Requests for favors by the patient, for example, to borrow a book from the analyst, must be declined. First, they must be declined because granting favors tends to put the patient in an inferior position. Second, and more importantly, acceptance would confuse the patient about the therapist's role, which is to analyze the patient's communications. The analyst must especially avoid engaging in actions which diminish the patient's autonomy or motivation toward self-responsibility.

From this point of view, it makes little difference what the patient asks of the analyst, as long as it is something other than analyzing; the analyst must decline to grant any and all such requests. Indeed, requests for advice, sleeping pills, intercessions with disturbed relatives, and even for sexual gratification fall in the same class. Each is a reasonable desire for the patient to have, and the analyst must certainly not discourage the patient from satisfying any such wish; but he must not satisfy any of them himself! Granting any such favors is "acting-out" on the part of the analyst, for, in so doing, he steps out of his role of analyzing and instead engages in a piece of "real-life" transaction with the patient.

To recapitulate: If the patient offers gifts and the therapist accepts them, the contract will become, as a result, overfulfilled. The patient may respond with efforts to compensate for this imbalance, for example, by wanting to reduce the fee or by trying to "get" more from the therapist. The therapist may respond, in turn, with some inappropriate (nonanalytic) gesture to mitigate his guilt for "taking" too much from the patient, for example, by prolonging the patient's session.

On the other hand, if the patient requests favors and the therapist grants them, the contract will become, as a result, underfulfilled. Both patient and therapist may then respond with efforts to compensate for this imbalance. In addition to these problems of over- and underfulfillment of the contract, participation in such extra-analytic activities with the patient confuses the analytic relationship by introducing into it unanalyzed (and often unanalyzable) "real-life" transactions between patient and analyst.

If the analyst conducts himself as an autonomous therapist, he avoids having to lay down prohibitions for the patient. It is, of course, essential that the analyst never assume the role of a forbidding authority. Such a posture would run counter to the basic aim of autonomous psychotherapy. Therapist and patient must not try to control each other's behavior; instead, each must influence the other by controlling his own conduct.

These principles are exemplified by the analyst's handling of the patient's wish to offer gifts or request favors. The therapist does not prohibit the patient from giving gifts; instead, he does not accept gifts and explains why. Similarly, he does not prohibit the patient from asking favors; instead, he does not grant them and explains why.

The Conditions Necessary for Contracting

As we have seen, contracting may fail if either party feels that he is much weaker or much stronger than the other. Like games, contracts require two nearly equal participants. In ordinary games, the players must be well matched in skill (though not necessarily in any other way). What corresponds to this in autonomous (contractual) psychotherapy?

It is neither expected nor necessary that patient and therapist be equal in their knowledge of psychology and their skill in conducting psychotherapy. What is expected is that they be approximately equal in their willingness and ability to assume responsibility for themselves and toward each other. This means that each participant must believe that he has something to give his partner and that in return he may make some legitimate demands on him. We cannot speak of negotiations and contracts unless we have two parties, each of which needs something and also has something to offer. The patient, for his part, needs and wants psychotherapeutic help; in return, he offers the therapist money and responsible cooperation in therapy. The therapist, on the other hand, needs and wants money and opportunity to do his chosen work; in return, he offers the patient analytic knowledge and skill. On this basis, meaningful negotiation and contracting can occur between them.

Negotiation is impossible or tends to break down whenever the bargaining position between patient and therapist is excessively unbalanced. The exploiter may feel that he has nothing to give or that the therapist has enough or too much and hence needs or deserves nothing from him. The exploitee may feel that the therapist is needy and hence must have whatever he demands or that he himself requires little and can therefore give others almost anything they wish. In either case, negotiations will falter. These considerations highlight the necessity for both patient and therapist to frankly recognize both what they need and what they offer each other in exchange.

I therefore find it difficult to imagine how contractual therapy could work without the patient's paying a fee to the analyst, for it is paying the analyst, more than anything else, that enables the patient to be a responsible, negotiating party to a contract with him. Similarly, the situation would be more complicated if the therapist did not need the patient's money. What could the patient give such a therapist? Of course, it is possible to do psychotherapy and to "help" a patient without the patient's paying the therapist for his services; but such therapy would be neither contractual nor, in our terms, analytic.

As in any bargaining situation, the contract between patient and therapist and their fulfillment of its terms may have one of three outcomes: it may be mutually advantageous and equally fair to both; the patient may exploit the therapist; or the therapist may exploit the patient. The autonomous therapist must aim, honestly and sincerely, at contracts that are not only mutually binding, but also mutually fair and gratifying. He can do this, on the one hand, by exerting his own efforts in this direction and, on the other, by informing the patient (in the appropriate context) of the dangers of unilateral exploitation and enlisting his vigilance against this hazard.

THE ANALYSIS OF LANGUAGE GAMES

In traditional psychoanalytic terms, the aim of much of analytic work is to help the patient gain access to his unconscious. In other words, analyst and analysand collaborate in rendering the (patient's) unconscious conscious.

Formulating the analytic enterprise in terms of communications, rule-following, and game-playing enables us to describe the process of analysis differently and, I think, more accurately. I have already indicated some of the work the analyst must do, for example, in translating the patient's messages from the language of needs into that of promises. I now want to expand on this theme by showing what is entailed in the analysis of language games.

In part, the patient's problem is that his aspirations and interpersonal strategies are disguised, not only from others, but from himself as well. He expresses himself indirectly, through suffering, symptoms, dreams, allusions, and so forth. The analyst's task is to help the patient make the inexplicit explicit, to communicate directly, rather than indirectly. To do this, a large part of the therapeutic work must be devoted to the analysis of language games. Although the games played by various persons vary greatly, certain categories of language game can be distinguished (for example, the languages of bodily symptoms, of unhappy personal relationships, of persecution). Indeed, we have here a method for transforming traditional psychiatric nosology into an operationally meaningful typology of personal conduct, in accordance with the predominant idiom the patient uses to express his problems of living.

The Language of Excuses and the Language of Responsibility

From the many language games that people play, I shall select two that are especially pertinent to the work of the contemporary psychotherapist. Much of the so-called psychopathology which the therapist tries to understand, decode, and translate into another idiom centers on the patient's attempts to evade responsibility for his aspirations, desires, feelings, thoughts, and actions. By "interpreting" (that is, by pointing out) the patient's evasions of self-responsibility and by refusing to assume responsibility for him, the analyst encourages and teaches the patient to accept and develop a more self-reliant attitude. Clearly, then, psychoanalysis is a *moral exercise* or, if one wishes to put it that way, a *moral therapy*. Because it deals with the nature and value of varying styles of personal conduct, it could not be anything else.

In the case we are now considering, patient and therapist are dealing with a pair of languages—the language of excuses and the language of responsibility. These correspond roughly to the person's self-experience as someone helpless and dependent on others (heteronomy), against his experience as someone capable and independent (autonomy). The former is characterized by the key expressions "I can't," "I must," "I had to," "I couldn't help it," and "I was ordered"; the latter, by the expressions "I want to," "I decided," "I chose," and "It was my fault." Some examples may illustrate the role of the analysis of language games in autonomous psychotherapy.

Let us begin with the case of the young student forced into a medical career by his father who complains of a work inhibition. He says: "I cannot study. What shall I do?" He is afraid (we need not be concerned here with the precise nature of his intrapsychic or interpersonal conflicts) to say to his father (and to himself): "I do not want to study medicine"; "I do not want to be ordered around by you." Instead, he *asserts himself* through the language of excuses; he thus achieves some of his aims and yet avoids responsibility for (some of) the consequences of his acts. This explains why so-called neurotic behavior is, in a very fundamental sense, "normal" as well as personally and socially useful and why it cannot and should not be changed by anyone but the patient himself. The patient will, however, change it only if he can act in a manner more satisfying to himself.

Here is another example. A young mother and housewife is dissatisfied with her life. She falls in love with another man, has an affair with him, and is contemplating divorce. She seeks help from a psychotherapist to whom she makes statements of this type: "Hard as I try, I am unable to love my husband. I can't continue my marriage." The therapist will encourage the woman to take more responsibility for herself and her life situation. She ought to be able to say (to herself and to such others as her analyst and her husband) to what extent she does not *want* to love her husband (who may not deserve her love) and does not *want* to stay married. The analyst assumes that, with clearer understanding of her wants, for both continuing and discontinuing the marriage, the patient will be in a better position to decide on the course of action she wishes to pursue.

The contractual nature of the analytic relationship makes it an ideal setting for effecting translation from the language of excuses into the language of responsibility. It is necessary, therefore, that the analyst assume responsibility for his part of the conduct of the analysis and that he not hide his acts and motives behind a screen of silence or of psychoanalytic excuses. At the same time, the analyst must challenge, tactfully but persistently, the patient's excuses. As the therapy progresses, many of these will be directed toward the analyst. The following example is illustrative.

A young man in analysis because of homosexuality is called up for military service. He says to the analyst: "My draft board wants me to get a statement from you about what is wrong with me." Note the linguistic form of the request; it is the draft board, not the patient, who asks for the expert opinion. The analytic task is to discuss who wants what and why and who is willing to do what and for whom. In other words, does the patient really want the analyst to give him a note? If so, what are the possible implications and consequences of such an act for the patient and for the analyst? What is the analyst's decision and his reason for it? What are the patient's alternatives?

Here is another example. A patient, chronically hypochondriacal and neurasthenic, cancels his analytic appointment because of illness. For such a person, feeling sick is necessary and reassuring. It is like a hoard of cash for an unscrupulous businessman. As the latter expects to bribe his way out of trouble, so the former expects to evade his obligations and difficulties by offering symptoms; he has learned that, like cash, illness is a widely accepted currency in human relations. He says to the analyst: "I am sorry I could not come, but I was too ill."

Here the task is to translate "I could not come" into "I did not want to come." This can be achieved only if the analytic situation is unlike most ordinary situations, where illness is a legitimate excuse. (It may also be in analysis, but not for individuals who play the illness game habitually.) The analyst must neither punish nor reward the patient for being ill. He can avoid doing this by explaining to the patient that he does not have to keep his analytic appointments if he feels disabled. At the same time, the analyst must remind the patient of the analytic contract which requires payment of a fee for each appointment, and he may invite the patient's suggestions for handling the fee for missed appointments. This sort of dialogue informs the patient that his illnesses, however unpleasant, are his responsibility, not the analyst's.

Next it is necessary to examine the consequences of various possibilities for both the patient and the analyst.

1. If the patient does not pay, he saves money and deprives the analyst of a fee he could earn from a nonhypochondriacal patient.

2. If he expects the analyst to accept his excuse as a valid one, he places the therapist in the position of either trusting or distrusting him; but the therapist's job is to analyze the patient, not to judge the authenticity of his excuse.

3. If the patient defers to the analyst's judgment of the severity of his complaints and hence the validity of his excuse, he places the therapist in the position of judging the patient's ability to attend the analytic session; but this is not the therapist's concern, and, if he makes it his, he will not be able to analyze the patient.

4. If the patient pays the fee whether or not he attends the session, his autonomy vis-à-vis the therapist remains intact, and the therapist can concentrate on the task of analyzing him.

In sum, the analysand's communications, framed in the language of excuses, must be systematically explored and decoded, and he must be invited to rephrase his messages in the language of responsibility. Thus, in addition to analyzing the transference neurosis, it is necessary for the therapist to cope with the patient's attempts to disregard the contract. He must be shown how he does this by interpreting his efforts to evade or change the contract. But this is not enough. Since the analyst is the second party to the contract, he must actually hold the patient to the terms of the agreement. The therapist who interprets the patient's contract evasions but at the same time permits them to occur becomes just another person with whom the patient re-enacts his habitual game-playing strategies.

14

The Terminal Period

How Does the Analytic Relationship End?

Let us begin with the sort of statement about terminating analysis and the sort of procedure for achieving it that I consider unacceptable. It is often claimed that psychoanalytic treatment may be discontinued, or ought to be, when the patient's transference neurosis is resolved. This is comparable to saying that a physician may stop treating a patient when his disease is cured. Both statements are tautologous; they simply assert that illness requires therapy, whereas health does not.

The typical, but incorrect, procedure for terminating analysis is closely related to this conceptual model of medical therapy. According to it, it is the therapist's responsibility to gauge his patient's progress in analysis and to decide when therapy should be brought to an end. But, as mentioned earlier, in agreeing to the analytic contract, the autonomous analyst relinquishes the power and the right to exercise this option (except for non-payment of fees or possibly as a sort of desperate self-defense against the patient's direct aggression). Thus, the decision to interrupt or discontinue a patient's analysis is in the same category as the decision to give him tranquilizers or electroshock treatments; they are moves that the autonomous psychotherapist is not permitted.

These, then, are ways in which analysis cannot and should not be terminated. How should it be? Because the patient must make the decision, the answer depends largely on the patient's personality and his relationship to the analyst. Indeed, the terminal phase of autonomous psychotherapy is likely to reveal the analysand's typical game-playing strategies and hence be useful for analytic work.

If, however, the analyst imposes his ideas about termination on the patient—for example, by trying to "wean" so-called dependent patients or by setting a date for termination—he will obscure the patient's contributions to this aspect of the encounter. In so doing, the therapist not only infringes on the client's autonomy, but also sacrifices important opportunities for analytic work. Indeed, just as the trial period may be the most significant part of the analytic encounter for some patients, for others it may be the terminal period.

It follows from this point of view and method that the analyst's contribution to the terminal period should not vary much from patient to patient, whereas the analysand's is bound to vary, depending on his personality and the problems he is trying to solve. It is therefore possible to make some generalizations about the analyst's conduct in the terminal phase, but not about the patient's; the analysand's contributions can only be suggested by illustrative examples.

The Analyst's Role in Termination

In a sense, preparation for termination begins at the onset of autonomous psychotherapy. As a rule, patients ask questions about the duration and termination of analysis almost from the moment they meet the therapist. Understandably, prospective patients are concerned, not only about what they are getting into, but also about how they can get out of it. Thus, the terminal period must be viewed in the context of the relationship that precedes it—the initial interviews, the trial period, and the contractual phase.

The therapist who follows traditional analytic technique, laying down rules for the patient to follow, will also wish to apply certain rules to govern termination. By the time analyst and analysand have traveled that far, the patient will expect to be instructed about the rules for termination and will be glad to follow them. On the other hand, if the analyst indicates that he wishes to preserve and enlarge the client's sphere of self-action and if he insists that all decisions—including starting, continuing, and ending analysis—are the patient's responsibility, the situation will be radically different. The client will not expect the analyst to tell him how or when to stop the analysis, but, on the contrary, will expect to decide this largely for himself.

This is not only an ideal; it is also a fact. It follows logically from the psychotherapeutic method. As a relationship progresses, the patient in autonomous psychotherapy realizes that the relationship is entirely his, to do with as he pleases. If he wants to continue it or end it at any time, he may do so, regardless of the analyst's opinion.

Of course, if a patient invites my opinion about termination and if I have one, I share it with him, as I would on any other matter that concerns him; and, if I do not have one, I share that view also. Thus, my patients and I have an understanding about the terminal period long before we come to it. When we do, it is subjected to the same scrutiny as is everything in the therapeutic relationship. As mentioned, the style of termination often reveals a great deal about the patient's typical social games and interpersonal strategies. The analysis of the terminal phase may thus serve as a summary of much of the analytic work that preceded it. In many instances, the patient himself can understand and analyze the terminal game.

EXAMPLES OF TERMINATIONS

In autonomous psychotherapy, the terminal period is likely to reflect the analysand's major life problem and his habitual or preferred mode of attempting to solve it. The following examples, in which identifying information is disguised, illustrate a few such themes.

Example 1: The Wish to Avoid Responsible Decision-Making

An internist was completing his analysis toward the end of the third year. We agreed on a termination date which fell a few weeks before the patient's departure for work in another city. Approximately two weeks before our last meeting, he reported the following dream:

> You were going on a vacation. You referred me to Dr. X. I said: "But that won't leave us any time for finishing." You said: "No, but we must stop anyway."

In the dream, the patient was surprised but not upset that I sent him away so abruptly. Dr. X was an organic-directive psychiatrist whom the patient considered the "last person" to whom he would turn for help. He suggested that the dream meant that he still hoped that I would "kick him out," as his father had never done. He would have preferred it if I, rather than he, had made the decision about termination.

The patient's father was very close to his only son—indeed, too close for the son's comfort. The father was always hovering about, ready and willing to help his son. Actually, he was "helpful" even when his son did not need help and would have preferred to be left alone. Thus, the patient had to emancipate himself from his father's protectiveness entirely through his own efforts. His complaint was that his father never encouraged him to be independent and self-reliant.

The analytic contract allowed a symbolic re-creation of what was partly a constraining, yet also a comforting, situation for the patient. By being endlessly available, the analyst behaved much as the patient's father had. The problem is not unusual; the analytic situation often resembles some aspect of the analysand's relationship to his parents. The only proper way to deal with this is to discuss and "analyze" it. This we did. Nevertheless, the patient kept hoping that I would "prove" that I was different from his father by "kicking him out." Had I decided on termination, I would have gratified his wish. Paradoxically, however, I would have only proved that I was *like* his father. In addition, we would have missed the opportunity to use the terminal phase, like all other parts of the therapy, for analysis.

Example 2: The Wish to Avoid Being Abandoned

A young man was preparing to end his analysis after approximately one year. He was afraid of all protracted relationships and significant commitments; thus, he was also afraid of analysis. Because of the divorce of his parents when he was a child, his significant early relationships always ended in a *surprising* way, usually unpleasantly for him. As he made plans to terminate, it became clear that he wanted to surprise me. He made several tentative plans to stop, changed them suddenly, and each time decided to continue therapy for another few months.

When I went along with his uncertain plans, he began to wonder whether he was hurting me by placing me in such an unpredictable position. (I felt that I had to accept these terms, since I had not specified before the contractual phase that I would have to be notified in a certain, definite way about termination. On the contrary, our agreement was, as usual, that the patient could come as long as he wanted to.)

Thus, the terminal phase, which occupied a considerable part of the analysis, was the most important in the entire therapeutic encounter. In it, the patient re-created many of the situations in which he was badly treated by his parents, but this time reversing the roles: he was the capricious parent; I, the child he had been.

Example 3: The Wish for Perfection and Permanence

The patient was a young woman, an only child. Her mother's overriding interest in life was to make life "safe and secure" for her daughter. Everything and everybody, especially the patient's father, was used, first by the mother and later by the patient herself, to serve this end.

As a result, the patient never emancipated herself from her mother, though she pretended that she had; this pretense made her feel adequate and helped maintain the fiction that she had a "good mother." In actuality, she never examined, never revised, and never brought to a meaningful, honest confrontation her relationship to her mother. Everything this patient did and every relationship she engaged in remained similarly incomplete and unresolved. She rationalized this through a strategy of perfectionism. Everything had to be "just so"; she kept working on her significant relationships, ostensibly hoping to improve them, but actually leaving them unchanged.

Her relationship to me became for her a "wondrous thing," which she was reluctant to bring to an end. The issue of termination was not even broached during the first four years of therapy, which lasted many more years. Its duration reflected this woman's deep-seated conviction that she was never quite ready to make a transition to a new activity, a new relationship, a new phase of life. Indeed, she dreaded change. It is significant that she began therapy with equal reluctance. She had considered doing so for more than a decade, but waited until the established pattern of her life threatened to disintegrate.

THE DURATION OF ANALYSIS

As a rule, the analytic relationship continues over several years. Many psychiatrists and psychoanalysts, including Freud, bewailed this fact and expressed the hope that, in due course, a more "efficient" and quicker analytic procedure would be devised. Like so many mistaken ideas about psychoanalysis, this also rests on the notion that analysis is a form of treatment for neurosis, comparable to medical treatment for, say, pulmonary tuberculosis. If this were so, it should be possible to improve analysis just as other medical treatments are improved, by mak-

ing it act more rapidly and effectively and by making it cheaper
and thus available to more people. However, to expect psychoanalysis to be "improved" in this way is to misunderstand the
nature of the analytic enterprise.

Psychoanalysis is not a medical treatment, but an education.
It is not like getting cured of a disease, but rather like getting
to know another person well or learning a foreign language or
a new game. How long does each of these take? It is with this
kind of human experience that analysis must be compared. Thus,
it can be understood why the analytic enterprise, by its very
nature, precludes speed. This does not mean, however, that, to
be useful, every analysis must last three, four, or more years.

There is another fundamental misunderstanding in the expectation that, with greater knowledge and skill, analysts ought to be
able to increase the speed of analyses. It lies in not realizing
that the duration of a particular analysis depends, neither on the
nature of the patient's "mental illness" nor on the efficiency or
inefficiency of the "treatment" used (though this plays a part),
but rather on the patient's needs and wishes to continue to
receive "analytic education."

Perpetual graduate students do not necessarily make the best
scientists nor always the worst. Conversely, students who drop
out of school early or who complete their education rapidly
may do much or little with what they have learned; some may
continue a process of self-education, whereas others may soon
forget whatever they have learned. The situation is similar in
psychoanalysis. Some analyses last long and ought to last long
because of the sort of person the patient is; others are and ought
to be relatively short. It is a grave mistake to link the effectiveness of analysis with its duration. In fact, the two are nearly
unrelated. Some persons learn more rapidly than others, whether
in school or in analysis. The same is true for analysts; some
work more quickly than others.

In sum, the duration of a particular analysis reflects two
things: the needs of the patient and the personal styles of

analyst and analysand as analytic game-players. We should expect this and not superimpose on analysis concepts and values alien to it. Only under such conditions can psychoanalytic treatment be an authentic and autonomous encounter between analyst and analysand.

Epilogue:

Advice to Therapists

Learning to Practice Psychoanalysis

I have argued that the analytic relationship is like a game, with analyst and analysand its players. This view of the analytic procedure has implications, not only for its theory and practice, but also for teaching it and learning it.

How do we learn to play games of skill and strategy? It is important that we be clear about the answer to this question, for what is true of games of this sort is also true of psychoanalysis. There are some things about games that can be taught and learned through the printed word and through didactic instruction; there are other things, however, that cannot and that must be acquired through practice.

What can be taught and learned formally are the rules of the game and the principles underlying the aim and structure of the game. I have tried to lay bare these two aspects of psychoanalysis. What cannot be taught and learned formally is *how* to play a particular game, in this case, how to be an analyst or an analysand. Indeed, it should be obvious that there are serious limitations to doing anything of this sort. After all, one cannot tell players how to play a game; that is their business. It is the very essence of games that the players are free to play or not and, within the rules of the game, to play as they see fit. If a person is coerced—either to play against his will or to play in a certain fashion—then he is no longer a game-player (in the ordinary sense); although such a player may appear to others as though he were playing a game, he will actually be "working," not "playing."

None of this is intended to deny that some ways of playing games are more effective than others. I merely wish to call attention to the crucial role of freedom in game-playing; a person whose moves in a game are regulated by others is considered a puppet or a robot. Players are ordinarily expected to be entirely free within the rules of the game. In keeping with this, a good player of almost any game will develop his distinctive style. How does this apply to the analytic situation?

Clearly, both analyst and analysand must be left free to conduct themselves as they see fit, as long as they keep within the rules of the analytic game. The competent analyst will thus develop his distinctive style of analyzing; this style is likely to vary somewhat from patient to patient and may also change as the analyst ages and is subjected to various experiences. The patient must, of course, be even freer to play the role of analysand as he sees fit than is the therapist to play the role of analyst. After all, the aim of the therapy is to observe and analyze the patient's game-playing strategies; if the analyst tells him how to behave, what is there to analyze? The value of the psycho-analytic situation lies in constraining the patient only slightly and in a general way, that is, by certain game rules only, rather than by demands for specific acts of compliance.

In addition to learning the rules and principles of autonomous psychotherapy, the therapist who wishes to become proficient in this activity must practice it. The beginning therapist may profit from "supervision" of his work if the relationship between him and his supervisor is also autonomous, that is, if the supervisor is the therapist's agent.

What about the therapist's personal analysis? Does it not help him to learn how to be an analyst? I have deliberately omitted discussion of this subject in earlier parts of this book and will not say much about it here.

I believe that it is generally helpful for the therapist to have a personal analysis, but let me add some qualifications. I have serious reservations about the value of coerced "training analyses," practiced in conformity with the requirements of the various psychoanalytic organizations. Though such an "analysis" may help the therapist gain accreditation, it is unlikely to help him become liberated from his inner constraints. Personal analysis, undertaken outside the jurisdiction of an organized training system, is more likely to be personally helpful to the therapist. But here, too, we ought to be sober about what to expect. Having a "good analysis" does not make one a good analyst, nor does knowing one's "blind spots" ensure him against analytic ineptitude.

In other words, I do not consider a personal analysis indispensable for competence in analyzing. Indeed, if the therapist's analysis is autonomous, it can have only one effect: to set him personally free to do what he wishes. Some analyzed therapists may want to practice autonomous psychotherapy; others may prefer to practice differently. The notion that the psychotherapist's personal analysis is bound to make him a better analyst than he would be without it is illogical and probably untrue.

What the analyst needs more than anything else is genuine interest in doing analytic work and a readiness to enter into a relationship with his client on the basis of well-considered principles, rather than with an amorphous therapeutic intent. If such a person has also had a period of analytic work and is thus familiar with the analytic game from the point of view of the analysand as well, so much the better.

There is one more type of instruction that can be useful to prospective game-players, namely, advice about some aspects of the game—in our case, about certain recurrent types of analytic situation. In conclusion, I shall offer some suggestions of this kind for those interested in practicing autonomous psychotherapy.

ADVICE TO THERAPISTS

Forget That You Are a Physician

If you are a psychiatrist, do not let your medical training get in your way. If you are not medically trained, do not secretly aspire to be a doctor. If the service you propose to sell is analysis, you owe it to your clients and to yourself to be a competent analyst. Competence in another discipline—for example, in medicine—is not an excuse for incompetence in the theory and practice of psychoanalysis.

You Are "Helpful" and "Therapeutic" if You Fulfill Your Contract

Do not feel that you must comply with the patient's requests for nonanalytic services. You are not responsible for the patient's bodily health; he is. You need not show that you are humane, that you care for him, or that you are reliable by worrying about his physical health, his marriage, or his financial affairs. Your sole responsibility to the patient is to analyze him. If you do that competently, you are "humane" and "therapeutic"; if you do not, you have failed him, regardless of how great a "humanitarian" you might be in other respects.

You Must Get to Know Your Patient

You must see the patient often enough and over a long enough period to get to know him well. There must be continuity in your relationship. To understand and master a new game, some players require more exposure to it than others. If you are a beginning therapist, you would do well to charge less and see your patient more often than you might otherwise. With your first few patients, have at least four weekly sessions and, if possible, five or six. If you see patients only three times a week, you may have difficulty following the moves in the game, and, if only twice a week, your chances of becoming a skilled autonomous psychotherapist are slim.

Do Not Let Yourself Be Coerced by "Emergencies"

If you have conducted yourself autonomously at the beginning of the treatment and have progressed satisfactorily to the contractual phase of the relationship, one of the major threats to the therapy is an emergency. Remember your contract, and do not be coerced by an emergency to abandon it. It is unimportant whether the emergency is real or whether the patient is testing you to see whether you will maintain your analytic role. (In any case, you will not be able to find out unless you do.) Here is an example. The patient, a homosexual, is arrested by the police. Do you intervene? No; this is a problem for the patient and his attorney.

If you intervene in an emergency, you engage the patient in another game and vitiate your usefulness as analyst. For instance, your patient may be depressed; you may want to hospitalize him and treat him with electroshock. In my view, this is like interrupting a bridge game to advise your partner on managing his business or getting a divorce. The advice may be good, bad, or indifferent, but it is not part of a game of bridge. In the analytic game, once you step out of it, you may find it difficult or impossible to get back in again. This is an important characteristic of contractual psychotherapy, and both you and your patient must recognize it.

Do Not Misconstrue the Patient's Feelings and Ideas about You

What the patient feels and thinks about you is as "real" as what anyone else feels and thinks. Though it may be reasonable to label some of his feelings and thoughts "transference," remember that, in doing so, conduct is being judged, not described. As a working hypothesis, assume that, in proportion as the patient is preoccupied with you as a person and as a source of approval and love, he is avoiding the responsibility for deciding what he wants to do with himself. He thus tries to solve the problem of having to give meaning to his life by attaching himself to the meaning you have given yours. You betray him if you encourage his doing so.

Your Life and Work Situation Must Be Compatible with the Practice of Autonomous Psychotherapy

If you practice autonomous psychotherapy, you will have to exhibit an attitude of "live and let live" toward your patients. It will be difficult for you to do this if you are coerced and harassed by others or if, outside your analytic practice, you engage in activities that require you to coerce and harass others. For example, if you are a resident in a state hospital or a candidate in an analytic institute, how will you be able to leave your patients alone when your superiors do not leave you alone? Will you be able to let your patients become freer than you are yourself?

Perhaps you will conclude that the only way you can be your own master is to be in full-time private practice. There is much to be said for this. Unfortunately, however, it is difficult to spend all one's time practicing analysis. If you see eight or ten patients day in and day out, the chances are that the level of your work may not be consistently high. A good solution to this dilemma is to combine analytic work with other activities compatible with it, for example, with teaching, research, or writing.

Do Not Take Notes

The psychoanalytic relationship is a personal encounter. You are not doing anything to the patient—at least no more than he is doing to you. You are not the observer and he the observed. Both of you play dual roles as participants in a relationship *and* as observers of it. What effect would note-taking have on your relationship with your mother, wife, or friend? Thus, do not be oblivious to the metacommunicative implications for the patient of your act of note-taking.

In any case, ask yourself why you want to take notes. To help you remember what the patient tells you? It will not do that, but *not* taking notes might. To record a case history? What will you do with it? To record material for research purposes? You can jot down what you think you will need after the interview or at the end of the day. If you are uncertain about the sort of thing you will need, notes will serve no purpose; a detailed account of the patient's "productions" is a useless document.

You Are Responsible for Your Conduct, Not for the Patient's

This is the central principle of autonomous psychotherapy. You are not responsible for the patient, his health (mental or physical), or his conduct; for all this, the patient is responsible. But you are responsible for your conduct. You must be truthful; never deceive or mislead the patient by misinforming him or withholding information he needs. Do not communicate about him with third parties, whether or not you have his consent to do so. Make every effort to understand the patient by trying to feel and think as he does. Finally, be honest with yourself and critical of your own standards of conduct and of those of your society.

In sum, you must be an analyst.

Index

DATE DUE

Demco, Inc. 38-293